SCARY
DIAGNOSIS

SCARY DIAGNOSIS

How I Took Charge of My Health and Life
and How You Can Take Charge of Yours

ALAN GELLER

With Hopes for
"Your" Best Possible Health!

[signature]

THREE RINGS PUBLISHING

Three Rings Publishing
Burlington, Ontario
www.threeringspublishing.com

Cataloguing in Publication Data available
from Library and Archives Canada

ISBN 978-0-9782748-0-1

Cover design: Angel Guerra/Archetype
Cover and author photo: John Rennison
Text design: Tannice Goddard/Soul Oasis Networking

Printed and bound in Canada by Friesens

This book is intended for biographical and informational purposes only. The
information contained in this book is not intended to substitute for informed
medical advice. You should not use this information to diagnose or treat a health
problem or disease without consulting a qualified health-care provider (for instance,
a qualified doctor, nurse, pharmacist/chemist, and so on). The author is not a doctor.
None of the individual contributors, publishers, editors, or anyone else connected to
this book can take any responsibility for the results or consequences of any attempt
to use or adopt any of the information presented in this book. Nothing in this book
should be construed as an attempt to offer or render a medical opinion or otherwise
engage in the practice of medicine.

To my wife,
Deborah Goodwin,
who was right there beside me, every step of the way.
There is an amazingly long list of people
who both love and respect Deborah.
Let this be a written record of the fact that my name
appears at the very top of that list

To my mother,
Sheila,
because a mother is a mother,
and she's mine

And to the memory of my grandfather,
Abe J. Geller — I miss you, Gramps

It's supposed to be a secret, but I'll tell you anyway.
We doctors do nothing. We only
help and encourage the doctor within.
— ALBERT SCHWEITZER

CONTENTS

PREFACE

I'm thrilled you have this book in your hands. It's the result of a lot of work. Writing a book, I now realize, is a lot harder than it looks. But it's also the result of something much harder for me than writing a book — receiving a totally unexpected and very serious diagnosis from my doctor after a life of "average" health and lots of energy.

I have put this book together to tell you my story of receiving the diagnosis, of the self-doubt and passivity that followed, and then of how I took charge of my own health and life, actually making my future look a whole lot better than what the professionals were predicting.

My hope and belief is that this book will bring you hope, give you support, and provide you with the tools and incentives you need to take action, if you or a loved one are going through a similar situation.

ACKNOWLEDGMENTS

PLEASE TAKE A MOMENT!

I must confess right here and now that for much of my reading life I skipped the acknowledgments section of almost every book I read. A couple of years back I decided to read through one and now I almost always do. I would certainly appreciate it if you would take the time to read mine. The folks mentioned below deserve not only my thanks but also your recognition.

My writing began as a solitary effort that turned into a team sport once I made the decision to self-publish. Working on the book was therapy for me — days on end of reading and writing, more or less alone (except for my wife, Deborah, and Zeke, the half-dog-half-little-person). The process of self-publishing was a whole different deal than writing. The result, for me as a writer and to some extent as a person, was sort of like a caterpillar becoming a butterfly. The outcome of all this was my scary diagnosis becoming *Scary Diagnosis* — this book. I'll leave it to you to decide whether this butterfly is one of those attractive ones people love looking at, or one of those scary ones they run away from screaming and waving their arms.

Almost every book owes its existence to a group or team of people. This one is certainly no exception. I am going to thank a bunch of people who helped me through this project in several different ways. Some may not even know they were a help and may be surprised to find themselves mentioned here.

Let's begin with the publishing team. I hired Arnold Gosewich as a consultant to help me through self-publishing after he was introduced to me by Dave Di Marcantonio from Instabook Canada. Arnold has such a long list of credentials, you need to do a search for him on the Internet to understand the breadth of experience and insight he offers. He helps would-be authors like me self-publish their material so we can maintain control of it and make it available in a "relatively" short period of time. He introduced me to Don Bastian (Bastian Publishing Services), whose professional eye was instrumental in achieving the clarity of the finished product you're about to read. Don and his team are consummate professionals and incredibly dedicated. Thanks, Don. Arnold also introduced me to Angel Guerra, a talented graphic artist who not only designed the cover but also read the original draft and gave me some much appreciated commentary. He in turn introduced me to Tannice Goddard of Soul Oasis Networking and together they did the all-important page design and layout. The cover photos were graciously taken by John Rennison.

Before the publishing team was formed, there was already a group of great people instrumental in one way or another in sparking this book. I'd like to start by thanking my brother-in-law, Brad Goodwin, and Anne Marie Enright, Jill Mills, and Jackie Truty, who have all worked with my wife and me for years in our business. My wife and I consider them family. Knowing they were and are there through the "illnesses" was and is a great comfort to me and a super support for my wife. They are that business! Thanks!

Lots of doctors were involved in my journey. Some of them are mentioned by name below or further into this book. Others are not, and I'm guessing after reading my thoughts they may prefer it that way. Whether or not I ultimately felt any one doctor, nurse, health-care provider of any flavor, or anyone else who tried to help me in any way was beneficial to my health and experience, they deserve my gratitude just for being there. I've learned in life that we are the sum total of our experiences, both good and bad. So, my thanks to anyone who came into contact with me "professionally" through my initial symptoms and ongoing health efforts. Tackling a health crisis can be a difficult and sometimes thankless job, and when things look bad, we patients really need you!

Five doctors deserve some extra special attention. First, Dr. Bernard Wolos, who is my family doctor and helped quarterback my game plan — all while going through stem cell treatments (using his own) himself for cancer. I am happy to report that the treatments were successful and he appears healthy and well today (a story unto itself).

Second, Dr. Brian Smuk. Poor Brian (or Brain, as I occasionally call him after several typing errors made it seem applicable) must have dealt with endless abuse as a kid because of his last name. No doubt a noble name but one that other kids probably couldn't resist. As a result he often uses just Dr. Brian to this day, even with adults. Dr. Brian spent endless hours with me working and talking through all kinds of issues. His interest and expertise resulted not only in our becoming good friends, but also in our opening a nutritional testing clinic together, the first of which is in Burlington, Ontario, and is called Applied Nutrition Canada Corp. The information he supplied to me through research and testing remains to this day part of what I rely on to make health and wellness decisions.

Third, Dr. Paul Cutler and his staff. Dr. Cutler is an out-of-the-box doc extraordinaire. I believe he should one day be recognized as a shining example for his methods of practice and patient care.

Fourth, Dr. Oksana Sawiak, a biological dentist and most certainly a visionary when it comes to the practice of modern dentistry. Dr. Sawiak and her staff and their office procedures should be studied by any smart and caring dentist looking for enlightenment or who otherwise happens to stumble upon this book.

Fifth, Dr. Glenn Sprague, a doctor of osteopathy, who has patiently taken the time and made the effort to understand what I'm going through and to offer both insight and treatment. Glenn is exceptionally good at what he does, even if it is hard to explain or understand.

In an effort to make sure you continue reading this, I will just list some folks quickly for this next bit. Margaret Lott was my initial proofreader and incredible pie maker (Lotts and Lots Tea Room); my sisters, Caren, Alice, Jane, and Catherine and their families, for their love and support; my cousin, Dr. Bob Geller; my old friend, Billy, known professionally as William N. Fords; Garrick Grayden, for checking up on me and being there; Robert (Rock) Marziano and Dave Di Marcantonio of Instabook Canada, for their support and wading through the first draft; Rick Claydon and Bryan Grenier at Stonegate Capital Management, for their ongoing advice; Kevin Mulcahy, an accountant who gets what's important in life, and his team; our Dinner Group — Ruth and Jim Roberts, Denise and Larry Teatero, and Nancy and Cam Playfair — who provide intellectual and spiritual stimulation, not to mention some good meals; Al Willick, for the same; and Bill Spicer and John Coppins (John called just as

I typed his name —weird). These last two, among others, tolerate my golfing efforts and provide much appreciated moral support.

Some additional folks are Dr. Wade Rafacz (way ahead of his time); Jim Poling, for his valuable time, input, and support; and Alexander Townsend (Jin Shin Do practitioner), who helped me and led me to Dr. Brian. In addition, Jackie Carey at Bulk Foods Warehouse in Burlington, Ontario, for her knowledge of supplements, Annie Van Alten at Dutchman's Gold, for her knowledge of local honey and bee products, and Gloria Aitken-Robertson, for taking such great care of us (including Zeke).

There were doctors and more doctors, so let's add to my list Dr. Paul O'Connor, Dr. Dana Hector, Dr. Evan Kaminer, and most certainly Dr. Bernard Bihari (the "father" of LDN). Special thanks to Jack Kuykendall, physicist and golf instructor (www.kuykendall golf.com), for taking the time to discuss golf, exercise, and nutrition with me.

My dedication acknowledges my wife and best friend Deborah Goodwin (Geller), but in case you skipped it, I'll just mention her again — she deserves the extra mention. I'll also make note of my stepfather, Noel Schwartz, who was helpful in ways he doesn't know, and my mother, Sheila, who was and is a tremendous influence on me.

No doubt there are all kinds of other people who should be mentioned here. If I missed you, please know you're part of the health and life I am enjoying today and you are appreciated. So please forgive me and consider yourself officially thanked!

Finally, I want to list my nieces and nephews. They can thank Jamie for this because when she found out I was writing a book she asked if she was in it. To be fair I'm listing all of them in alphabetical order: Adam, Ashley, Brian, Brittany, Jack, James, Jamie, Jason, Nolan, Rebecca, and Sam.

No self-respecting dog lover can leave their "second best friend" out of their acknowledgments section, so here it is: thank you, Zeke. At this very moment he's nudging me (spooky and weird) — I'm guessing he wants out!

INTRODUCTION

WHO SHOULD READ this book?

- Anyone who has received a scary diagnosis of their own.
- Friends and loved ones of those who have received a scary diagnosis.
- Anyone who thinks they or someone close to them will eventually receive a scary diagnosis.

I figure that includes pretty much everyone on the planet.

The focus of this book is personal. It is my story. It's about how I received sobering news from a doctor and how I took charge of my health and life in the aftermath of that news. And it's your story, too. My belief is that as you read my story, you will be comforted — which is very important — but motivated, as well, to take charge of your situation. I also include practical information that will help you in your own research and in your own interactions with health providers.

For much of this book I speak to readers as if they are patients, the ones with the scary diagnosis. For anyone else reading this book, please understand that what I have to say to patients will give you valuable insight into what they are going through and how to help and support them. You will be doing a wonderful thing for them by motivating them to be proactive — to be active participants in all aspects of the health and life choices they are facing.

I have experienced a scary diagnosis in two different ways. The first was through observing a loved one go through hers. This may be more difficult than having the problem yourself — at least it often seems that way, especially at the beginning. My wife has been diagnosed with cancer twice, and beat it both times. In these situations you, the observer, are called on to be "the strong one," whereas in fact the helplessness you're feeling as a spectator can be a major part of the problem. Just when you need to be optimistic and supportive, your lack of focus, feeling of shock, or even state of depression can make you more of a liability than an asset. But don't worry. This book will provide you with both insights and tools to help you handle this situation.

The second way was through my own, more recent scary diagnosis, which provides the "story" part of this book.

Having played both roles has certainly rounded out my views of illness and health.

Patients and non-patients alike will benefit from some of the research I've done, and from following my lead and doing their own research. The goal is for all of us to get information that will help us understand both what's really happening and the background for decisions that need to be made. In my case, my wife was a tremendous help and support as she patiently made all kinds of efforts to understand what I was going through. This put her in a great position to discuss alternatives with me.

In what follows I won't be giving a lot of detailed information about any individual illness, disease, or condition. I'd rather help you learn how to proceed on your own — how to chart your own course. I'll also remind you regularly why it's important — no, essential — to be proactive and to take control of your own situation. You need to become what I have come to call "productively proactive."

I am not a doctor. I am a patient. I am not anti-doctor or anti-pharmaceuticals. In fact, I believe you need to leave no stone unturned, exploring every option, getting as many opinions as possible, investigating as many potential causes and treatments as you can. Doctors and medical advice have been a key part of my team and strategy, and they need to be part of yours, too.

This book didn't start out as a book. Once I finally received my diagnosis and got past my initial emotional shock and awe, I started to talk to, and tried to help, other people who had received or were receiving their own diagnoses. The more I learned about illness, health, and wellness, the longer these conversations took. I had to start writing some basic stuff down because I was overloading people with too much information. I'd email what I wrote to the people who called me, telling them to "read this and call me in the morning."

Finally I realized that putting my story and this information between two covers made more sense, and they became the book you're holding in your hands right now.

Here's where we're going to go together. The book moves from the story of my scary diagnosis to advice about going through the diagnostic process, about dealing with personal issues, and about understanding the healthcare process. It also deals with how you can research your condition, mainly on the Internet, and examines lifestyle and alternative medicine issues. I also present two unusual case studies, one on LDN and the other on dentistry. The book concludes with a word on personal renewal — not just mine but yours as well.

My hope is that my story and my advice — as one who has been there, and is still there — will comfort you and inspire you to take action. Being in control of your own health is very empowering, even in the face of your very own scary diagnosis.

ONE

I HAVE *WHAT*?

Where ignorance is bliss, `tis folly to be wise.
— THOMAS GRAY

BEFORE I HAD any serious thoughts about "sickness" or of ever needing a diagnosis, I saw myself as somewhat of a plain vanilla type of guy. I grew up with my mother, stepfather, and four sisters. Until I was seven years old or so I shared a room with my older sister in a two-bedroom apartment in a beachside suburb of New York City (yes, there are such places). After that I slept in a tiny den, until I was 13 years old. I figure we were your basic lower middle to middle class family, in what was then a quiet and mostly middle class neighborhood. Being the product of a divorce, I did the visitation thing, spending most Sundays with my father and "his" family in New Jersey.

When I was about 13 we moved to a house that needed tons of work. It wasn't far from where we lived but was in a much more upscale part of town. We were "moving on up."

My stepfather was proving to be successful not only in business but also, as a hands-on kind of guy, in do-it-yourself renovations. I worked with him on the house, which resulted in a relationship that has become more like a friendship, one I truly value.

My mother is a wonderful person. She is over a decade past a major bypass operation and doing well. I call her every Monday and have for as long as I can remember. My sisters are, for the most part, healthy, and three of the four remain married with kids. One is divorced with no kids and seems to be doing fine.

I think you'll agree that my childhood was "average" for someone my age "graduating" from a divorce. In some ways my family was somewhat dysfunctional. But I think most people, if asked, would describe their own families that way. Based on what I now know about what others from divorced homes have experienced, I am thankful for how things have turned out. I'm also grateful for my family and friends and what I've been able to achieve in life.

I was a mediocre student with grades to match. I was born in 1955, so I was a teenager during the final years of the Vietnam war. I took part in many of the things that happened during that time, including smoking pot, playing Frisbee, and surfing. I was pretty good at the first two, but not so much at the third.

If you're wondering, yes, I did inhale.

I liked fishing, and still do. I had a super group of friends as a teenager, after being somewhat of a loner as a kid. I remain close to some of them today, even though we rarely see each other. I had my first job at 14 and have worked pretty hard, with occasional exceptions, ever since.

I had thoughts of becoming a teacher. Given my grades and my family's financial constraints, I was fortunate to be able to attend the

State University of New York at New Paltz for a year. It was great, but mostly party time.

My stepfather, skeptical about future options and my earning potential as a teacher, was concerned he might have to support me if I didn't get my act together and choose a "better" career: a sad commentary on the state of teaching that is still accurate more than 30 years later. After that first year he opened a newspaper and asked me, based on the salaries and numbers of jobs listed, what I wanted to be (very clever).

After rejecting the idea of being a doctor or lawyer (I wasn't big on blood and the law involves way too much nonsense), I said I thought engineering might be the ticket. It seemed about right for my skills, even though my grades had been marginal for most of my academic career. I had always been vaguely interested in the sciences, and loved science fiction. I had done well that first year at college, grade-wise, and math and science seemed to be clicking for me. This was surprising considering my often-altered states of consciousness at the time.

I changed my residence to New Jersey, where my father lived, and miraculously got into Rutgers University School of Engineering. After struggling through the first two years, when many students are weeded out, I got the hang of it and graduated two years later with a B.Sc. in civil and environmental engineering. I moved almost immediately to Atlanta to take a pretty good job in environmental work.

After I'd spent six or so years of working mostly at power plants, the company I toiled for was purchased by a Fortune 500 company and imploded shortly thereafter. Being independent and always convinced I could do things better than others, I wanted to try my hand at working for myself. I moved back to my parents' house because the business I was buying — a sort of luncheonette and general items store, which I imaginatively named The General Store — was in my childhood neighborhood.

After a year and a half of seven-day work weeks, trying to keep my business (and the building it was in, which I had also purchased) standing, I sold both and went back to engineering. For a brief period I did so as a consultant. I lived in Hoboken, New Jersey, with my cousin, Bob (who's like a brother to me), and traveled to the southern states and Texas regularly. Hoboken was fun and convenient — being close to Newark airport was a major plus. But I still wanted to work for myself, so I began looking for another business opportunity. I have always been pretty frugal, so I was saving some money, adding it to the modest amount I had made selling the business and building. Traveling a lot for work leaves little time for much else, so that also helped me save.

I ended up looking into a franchise opportunity in warehousing and selling cosmetics, something I found through a friend, and was instead hired by the parent company to work corporately, with the understanding that my primary interest was to eventually own a franchise. I moved to Valley Forge, Pennsylvania, and within less than two years "purchased" a franchise. (The way they worked it out was to cut my pay and offer me the franchise option as part of my compensation.) I went into business with the woman who would become my wife. She was from Hamilton, Ontario, a city located between Toronto and Niagara Falls. We moved to Long Island, New York, to open the business.

After we had built and operated that business for more than a year, my wife became homesick. I had met her through the business, and she also owned and operated a similar and successful franchise in Canada. She was traveling back and forth monthly, which can be tough in a lot of ways. So we sold the franchise in Long Island and moved close to her hometown, where I began working in my wife's business with her, her family, and a fantastic staff (whom we consider family).

It's now almost 20 years later. In addition to the franchise, we have owned and operated a couple of other small businesses, some successful and some not, and again worked corporately for our franchisor, running the Canadian operation. All in all we have done quite well, but it took a lot of hard work, and both of us have paid the price health-wise.

When I went through the attack that resulted in my diagnosis, beginning on February 5, 2004, I was looking into a couple of new business ideas. One was in the health and wellness field and stemmed from my wife's bouts with cancer. Preparing for this new business turned out to be good timing; I had little to do with the day-to-day running of our franchise and had cleared away most of the other things that would have taken up my work time.

My wife and I have no children, by choice. I was 33 and she 30 when we married. This is, for both of us, our first and only marriage. Call us selfish, but we both came from families with lots of kids (five and six, respectively), and both of us ate lots of spaghetti, potatoes, and meatloaf growing up. My wife is a smart and caring woman with a vibrant spirit, and we were both enjoying the life we were making for ourselves. We love dogs, and I'd like to say here and now that we have the best damn dog in the world. He's a Yellow Lab and his name is Zeke. (Sorry, I couldn't resist.)

Before all this, I had been relatively healthy and certainly was very active. I had been in a hospital only once, to have a fish hook (the dreaded treble hook) removed from my forearm. (Don't laugh — it's easier than you think to hook yourself, and hard to get them out.) I had some dental and related mouth issues, but no other operations or broken bones. Knocking out an eyetooth playing touch football has plagued me for years, but compared with what many people have experienced by the time they hit midlife, things had gone pretty well for me.

THE END OF LIFE AS I KNEW IT

And so it began. On a Wednesday two days after my 49th birthday, I woke up and noticed that the vision in my left eye was a little fuzzy. I thought maybe I had slept in a weird position. The next day things appeared to be a bit fuzzier. It seemed the change in my left eye was making things look brighter, but with less contrast.

I called my optometrist for an appointment. He fit me in the next day because I had been diagnosed with central serous retinopathy (CSR) in that eye some years back. CSR sounds bad, but it was just a condition in which a bit of fluid had leaked in the back of my eye, causing a slight distortion in my vision. It was frightening at the time, but had cleared up for the most part. After about a year of having CSR, however, it seemed that, as far as my left eye was concerned, I was seeing the world through a tiny bubble. I barely noticed it just before this new problem. It's interesting and important to note that CSR is one of the many, many conditions that have no clearly defined cause, based on our current knowledge. That last sentence is very important. You may want to reread it.

Was the CSR somehow related to this new fuzziness? No one knew for sure then, nor do they know to this day.

It was now Friday — day three — a very bad day of the week to have a health-related problem, I discovered, because most of the people you may need to see on the weekend will be off work. Try to never get sick on Friday (unless, of course, you're really skipping out on work).

My optometrist concluded I had about a 15–20% loss of vision in my left eye. The problem was not so much focusing as processing light and color. He suspected, given my history, that it might be CSR again, although he didn't actually see anything to confirm his suspicions.

I told him the symptoms were nothing like the original bout of CSR, which was the kind of comment I was going to repeat regularly for countless days to come.

He told me he thought it shouldn't get much worse over the weekend and scheduled me for additional testing on Monday. Wrong!

Saturday brought pain and pressure behind my left eye, and decreased vision. I hadn't slept well. My vision was about a third gone in that eye.

I was scared and stayed home waiting for Monday. By now I was doing a lot of pacing.

On Sunday my vision was about half gone, and I was panicking.

I went to a university-affiliated hospital nearby and signed into the emergency room. I figured going to this type of hospital would be smart if it turned out that something out of the ordinary was happening to me.

Four hours later I saw an ER doctor. I could read about two-thirds of the eye chart, but I really couldn't see as well as that test indicated. I felt the results were misleading.

I had additional pain and pressure behind my eye and in my head. Some of this could have been from stress and lack of sleep, but clearly something was very wrong.

I was sent for an x-ray, which revealed what appeared to be a fairly severe sinus infection. I had suffered from sinus infections for years and had been on antibiotics, steroids, and other stuff, with little success. This could explain the pain and pressure, but didn't seem to be related to my eye.

The doctor was visibly concerned and told me he was going to contact the ophthalmologist on call. An ophthalmologist is like a more serious optometrist. Many of them perform surgery. I could see the doctor in an office, arguing on the phone. He was not happy when he returned; the ophthalmologist on call had refused to come in. It seems he was having his Sunday dinner and felt, given my history of CSR and my seeming sinus infection, that he didn't need to see me in person. He suggested, via the ER doctor, that I go to my regular ophthalmologist the following day. I was put on an antibiotic (this will be significant later) and told to stop at a drugstore on the way home to buy an over-the-counter decongestant.

I knew deep down the eye problem was probably not CSR. I was scared and submissive. I was also skeptical about more or different antibiotics doing much to help me, because they had never really handled my sinus infections in the past.

I was told I was being released.

The ER doctor was clearly uncomfortable with this and told me, if things got worse, not to waste time waiting for an appointment with my regular ophthalmologist but to come back to the ER the next day.

On Monday morning I noticed a further decrease in my vision. By now, five days in, I had lost about 75% of the vision in my left eye.

I was terrified. I tried to call my ophthalmologist, but his office wasn't open on Mondays. I didn't want to go back to the ER because of the long wait, and I was angry that I had not been kept there overnight. My wife remained calm on the outside, but I could tell she was way past panic on the inside.

I did end up going to the ER, because there was simply no other choice. After another four-hour wait I saw another doctor (of course not the same one as the day before) and explained everything that had happened.

He was professional, but appeared to be angry that I had been sent home Sunday night given my condition and all the unanswered questions. He seemed particularly upset that the ophthalmologist on call hadn't come in to have a look at me. That made four of us now who were frustrated with the great man who couldn't be bothered: two ER doctors, my wife, and me.

He also didn't believe (based on his observations and the ER doctor's notes from the previous day) that my eye problem was sinus-related or CSR-related.

My condition was degenerating very quickly and he was concerned. I could read only the top three lines of the chart with my left eye, wearing my glasses. My thinking was muddled. I was scared and confused. The pain in my head was worse. Unbeknownst to my wife and me, although it was now Monday (usually the best day to have a health issue because you have the whole week to take action before the weekend), it was some kind of doctors' holiday and yet again no ophthalmologists were in the hospital. Unbelievable, but true. The on-call ophthalmologist — again a different doctor from the previous day — also wouldn't come in. He, too, based on a telephone conversation, assumed I had CSR and a sinus problem.

My head was a mess. I was in pain, my brain was tingling, and I couldn't think straight. Having had many sinus infections, and prior experience with CSR, I was sure something else was wrong — very wrong! But what did I know? I was only the patient.

The ER doctors were worried and trying to help. Their concern was obvious. No one else seemed at all interested. This second ophthalmologist, though on call, was fully booked at his office and leaving for vacation the following day. However, he finally agreed to see me at his office if I was willing to wait till he was finished with everyone else.

I had a feeling the ER doctor must have threatened him. Regardless, I was off to see him.

My wife was doing all the driving because I was well past being able to do that safely. After two more hours of waiting — so much for any illusions we had about being considered a priority based on my status as an emergency from the ER — it was finally my turn.

The ophthalmologist did a thorough exam and concluded that my eye problem was probably not CSR. Although he was concerned, he wanted to hand me back to my family ophthalmologist. He then scheduled an angiograph (a process in which dye would be injected into my arm and my eye would be photographed). This was supposed to definitively confirm or eliminate CSR as a diagnosis. I had gone through this before when I did have CSR. The test was scheduled for Wednesday, so I had a day to wait.

Evidently, in our region, this test was done only on Wednesdays. Who knew?

SLOW TIME, HARD TIME

Waiting is very hard when you're panicking — it feels like a giant hypodermic needle is sucking strength and hope directly out of your body. In some ways it can feel worse than the symptoms that brought you to this state in the first place.

It was now Wednesday, February 11, a week since I woke up with a fuzzy left eye. A new eye doctor performed the angiograph and thought it might be CSR, given my history, but said it would be an unusual case in view of the test results and his examination. There was some discussion about my description of the symptoms and whether they could even be indicating CSR.

I was unable to see sources of light — nothing at all. Riding down the street at night was a bizarre experience. I couldn't see headlights or streetlights, or any point that was the source of light; all I saw was a void where the source of light should be. Everything else was way too bright. It was kind of like something you'd see in a science fiction movie or a special effect in a video game. As I mentioned, I like science fiction, but I can assure you I wasn't liking this at all.

I started to convince myself that my condition must be some weird kind of CSR. No one was offering any other choices.

I was scheduled for a second angiograph the following Wednesday. That meant seven more days of waiting. I needed to believe someone had a clue about what was happening to me. At this point I had no choice but to simply wait and count the days down.

Until now I was secretly concerned that whatever was happening to my left eye might happen to my right one as well, which would leave me basically blind. This gave me a sense of urgency to find out what was happening. If knowing what was happening meant treating me and possibly saving my vision, even in just one eye, I wanted to know *now*. The good news was that CSR typically doesn't affect both eyes, so I was actually hoping it was the culprit.

Although I had little indication, symptom-wise, of the apparent "massive" sinus problem that had shown up on the x-ray before the pain in my head set in, I had lived with sinus problems for so long that I considered how I felt to be normal. (As far as I am concerned, "normal" is a relative term, so we're talking normal for me.)

In addition to setting up a second angiograph, this new doctor thought I should see my family doctor for a referral to a neurologist. He didn't think my problem was neurological. I recall he said something like there was one chance in a hundred that it was, but that it was best to rule it out.

I had already decided to see my family doctor to enlist his aid in managing the information from all these other doctors, and to get his read on what might be happening to me. I called for an appointment.

After a couple of dropped calls on my cell phone (no doubt you can relate), I finally got through. I must have sounded crazed (the dropped calls didn't help), because they said to come over immediately.

My doctor's willingness to take me so soon not only shocked me but actually started me shaking.

My family doctor is an old-fashioned, level-headed general practitioner. I explained all that had transpired and gave him the note from the doctor who had administered the angiograph and had suggested I see a neurologist and get a CT scan as soon as possible. My doctor got on the phone personally — that's right, personally — and booked an appointment for me with a neurologist for the next afternoon. Given wait times to see specialists, this was a miracle. It should have calmed me down. But his personal attention and the priority booking actually ramped my level of concern up another notch. I figured I must be "nearing the end" to be getting this kind of attention.

He also booked an emergency CT scan for the next morning. Another miracle and another click up the anxiety scale.

He was clearly not happy with or impressed by what had happened to me thus far. He was angry about the way my case had been handled by his peers, or perhaps the "system" in general. It was hard to tell which.

GETTING SOMEWHERE

Interestingly enough, I noticed I "felt" much better. I felt something positive was happening. Someone other than my wife and me not only was concerned but also was taking action — real, substantive action. We had a plan and we were on the move.

After an unexplained two-hour delay in getting the CT scan done at the hospital (a different hospital from the one with the ER I had gone to), we rushed over to the neurologist's office to make our appointment on time.

He did an exam and called for the CT scan results. They actually already had the results — I was really impressed with that, but, if possible, even more nervous as a result of this astounding level of service. The long and frustrating sessions at the ER were still very fresh in my mind.

Nothing obvious popped up, yet he seemed suspicious. So was I. The CT scan did appear to confirm a whopper of a sinus infection. He wanted an MRI done and also an evoked potentials (EV) test performed as soon as possible. Not wanting to waste another minute, we agreed to have the EV test done immediately if it could be scheduled. As you might suspect, my wife and I were by now on red alert.

I believed that the neurologist had found something. I was certain, at the very least, that he suspected something, especially after he agreed to see me again the next day.

This fast service was offered only if I could get the EV test done immediately. We went back to the original hospital for the test, because they had a spot open. In the midst of all this, I was encouraged that things were moving, but worried that I was going to be the very last to know anything about what was happening to me and that the news was not looking good.

The EV test consisted of having electrodes stuck to my head and watching some graphics on a computer screen. The test measures the time it takes for nerves to respond to stimulation and, typically, the intensity of that response. Based on what I was seeing — or, more accurately, not seeing — I knew we were zooming in on the problem, and it certainly wasn't CSR.

The next morning was Friday the 13th. (Other than its being another Friday, which as I mentioned is a problem in and of itself, the fact that it was the 13th meant nothing to me.) I was the neuro's first appointment. He had the EV results and clearly knew something, but wouldn't tell us what he was thinking. He said he couldn't say anything until an MRI was done.

Around here that could be a one-month wait.

I agreed to do whatever it took to get an MRI done soon, even if it meant flying somewhere — though that prospect wasn't at all attractive to me, given how I felt generally and how my head felt specifically.

Plus, what about that "massive sinus infection"? Flying and sinus infections, especially massive ones, don't mix.

The neurologist's secretary called a local hospital. They said they could fit me in for an MRI on an emergency basis during the next three working days (weekdays and not holidays). I knew I was close to a diagnosis and didn't want to waste another minute. I also knew something bad must be happening, because everything and everyone had taken on a sense of urgency.

The neurologist also sent me for some blood tests. These were the first ones ordered by anyone since my problem began. I found this odd at the time and find it even odder now.

I had scheduled another appointment with my family doctor for that Friday afternoon. He was very concerned about me and wanted an update from my perspective. He also wanted to help me plan any additional steps.

By now I had lost about 95% of the sight in my left eye. During my visit with my family doctor, he scheduled an appointment with an ear, nose, and throat specialist (ENT) for Monday. She would have a look at my sinus problem. He added a nose spray to my medications and changed the antibiotic, because the one I was taking seemed to be ineffective, given the pain and pressure in my head. It was yet another very long weekend.

I took the medications and tried to stay calm. The vision in my left eye was basically zero. I could see shapes. Everything was super bright. Reading wasn't much fun, and it was tough to watch TV.

I put a patch over my eye like a pirate. That calmed my vision, and me, down a bit. Sometimes it's a good thing to be a pack rat; I happened to have a patch in our medicine chest from my bout with CSR. My head really hurt and it was "buzzing" more than ever. In addition to the panic and fear, I felt just plain lousy.

I was watching the clock with my non-patched eye, waiting for Monday.

Monday, Monday.

ONE STEP FORWARD, TWO STEPS BACK

A visit to the ENT doctor was next. The results were confusing. She saw no signs of a sinus infection. But both the x-ray and CT scans had seemed to indicate "definitively" that I had an infection, and the "infection" had been represented to me as an absolute fact by several doctors. Till now it was pretty much the only thing the doctors had claimed to know for sure.

I had been prescribed two different antibiotics and a nose spray, plus the hospital had told me to stop that first day on the way home to buy an over-the-counter decongestant. Stopping to buy decongestants was one of the last things I had felt like doing that day. It turned out it was also one of the last things I needed to do.

I was really hoping I did have a sinus infection. That, as the cause of the pain behind my left eye, was preferable to something more serious. It didn't feel like a sinus thing, but, once again, I was just the patient. That pain behind my eye was radiating to my ear and the back of my head. I was "tingling" and my mental capacity was certainly somewhat impaired.

The ENT doctor concluded I might have a very minor infection in one or more of my unreachable sinuses, but she didn't see any signs of a "massive" one. (She was using a little scope to have a look — I'll spare us both the details.) But she was certain that I had polyps. Nasal polyps are small growths inside your nasal passages or sinuses. She didn't think the polyps or any possible infection were affecting my eyesight. At least that was something the doctors all seemed to agree on, but it didn't seem like good news to me. Actually, it wasn't good news at all, because my eyesight was my primary concern and any sinus-related cause should have meant it would be relatively easy to fix.

She recommended I have an operation to remove the polyps when I was feeling better. Did she really need to be going there at this point, I wondered, given the mystery we were all supposed to be so desperately trying to solve (you know — my going basically blind in one eye in five days)?

I had read about this polyp procedure before, because other doctors through the years had suspected polyps to be part of my sinus problem. I knew that removing them didn't address the cause and was potentially a scary operation. Polyps often come back after being surgically removed. I didn't like the risk-reward picture. The operation, at one point, was described to me as basically "peeling my face off" in order to do a thorough job of removing the polyps. These days there are apparently less intrusive methods in most cases. Either way, the operation happens way too close to the eyes and brain for me to have been comfortable with it. Although polyps tend to block or irritate one's sinus passages, they are rarely a more serious problem than that. I should note that polyps do appear on the very long list of things that no one seems to know the cause of.

This proposed operation was the last thing I needed to be thinking about, given what was happening to my eye and head, and I figured it was best to put off even contemplating it for a later date (like probably never).

I often wonder why doctors don't pay more attention to what they're saying. Do they not understand the impact of their words on patients and their families? Sometimes it seems they are so focused on their specialty and how it relates to the patient at hand, they forget why the patient came to see them to begin with.

A very specific example of a doctor making a careless comment occurred when my wife was diagnosed with malignant melanoma. She had a mole removed from her leg by our family doctor and it proved to be malignant (proclaimed a hundred to one shot). During her first visit to an oncologist (cancer specialist), he informed her that malignant melanoma can be very dangerous and aggressive. He then said if it has spread you probably have five years or less to live. He actually said exactly that! Naturally, it was game over for my wife and panic for me. Incredibly, this was before any testing had indicated it had spread, which thankfully it had not. Why can't all doctors (some are extremely patient-sensitive) choose to talk about "best case," saving the doom and gloom for if and when it's necessary?

Actually, I've come to believe that regardless of how grim things look, the patient must maintain a positive attitude. My family doctor, when giving us the initial news on the mole, had been way more positive, assuming he had caught it in time and things would be fine.

This same lack of attention to who is saying what to whom and when happens with kids all the time. This is not only the case with some doctors but with adults in general. Kids are like sponges and they are *always* listening. Extra special care about what a child hears is necessary whenever a scary diagnosis is involved. Adults need to watch what they say and carefully monitor what health care professionals say to or in front of children. If something unnecessarily upsetting or confusing is said, adults need to be ready for immediate damage control.

Be that as it may (a phrase I have always loved and have been anxiously waiting to use), the ENT and polyps actions are still on hold.

Thinking back, was it any wonder that the antibiotics and decongestants I was pumping into myself weren't working? They certainly weren't helping me feel any better. In fact, I've never liked the feeling I get when taking decongestants.

Tuesday was another day of pacing around the house.

On Wednesday a second angiograph was done. I was already scheduled for the procedure, so I kept the appointment, hoping CSR would be magically confirmed and end this Groundhog Day nightmare. (You know — reliving stuff over and over without resolution.) Just as a point of interest, Groundhog Day also happens to be my birthday.

I can tell you that the angiograph was painful. Having flash photography done of your eye while it's propped open with a brace and dilated with drops (have a look at a similar scene in the movie *A Clockwork Orange*) is no fun.

The results were again inconclusive. I was getting a bit crazed. This test was supposed to be conclusive — it was the "definitive" test for CSR. The doctor felt any CSR leakage must be across the "black" center of my eye and therefore not readily visible. He was basically at a loss and wanted to schedule me to come back in a month.

Things all of a sudden felt like they were drifting out of control, and I was getting really pissed (as in angry).

SLIPPING THROUGH THE CRACKS

Meanwhile, I had been waiting for a call from the hospital to schedule the MRI of my head.

An MRI, like a CT scan and an x-ray, is a way to get a picture of what's going on inside you, detecting additional detail regarding soft tissue — in my case, my brain.

I hadn't heard from the hospital as promised and felt things were taking too long. I was getting pretty negative.

I didn't want to be a labeled as a problem patient by being a pest, but I called the hospital about the MRI anyway. They told me I had "slipped through the cracks." I wasn't on the schedule at all. They couldn't even find my file. I was courteous but frantic on the phone. The nurse took pity on me and scheduled me for 8:30, Wednesday evening. There is typically someone who can fit you in somewhere for almost anything. The trick is getting them to relate to you as a person and take your case on as a priority.

An MRI of your head is an unpleasant experience — at least it was for me. My body was strapped to a table and my head was stuck in a metal frame to hold it still. The table, with a surrealistic hum, slid into a tunnel. I was asked to stay perfectly still as the machine buzzed (as if my head wasn't buzzing enough) and whirred for almost an hour. I was shaking when I got out of the tunnel. It is very confining and makes pretty much everyone feel claustrophobic.

There was a mirror above my eyes angled so I could see the operators in the control room during the procedure, and I'd been handed a panic button, which was supposed to help me keep calm (yeah, right!).

Calm I was not. I never opened my eyes once in that tunnel, not once. I focused all my thoughts, the best I could, on each and every breath I took. I needed this procedure and was willing to do almost anything to get through it and find out what was happening to me. From this and other experiences, I've come to believe the desire to be a model patient is a "normal" tendency early in an illness. I've discovered it's very common for patients, especially early in the diagnostic process, to think they'll somehow be rewarded for their submissive participation, perhaps with the news it was all a big mistake and they're fine.

You don't get the results from your MRI until you go back to see the doctor who ordered it.

This was a bit frustrating because I could see the pictures of my head (the inside of my head, that is) as I left the MRI area. They were displayed in living color on several computer screens.

Sleep was very tough, but thankfully my doctor had prescribed a mild sedative. It barely worked, but it was better than nothing. Sleep is even more important than normal when you're facing a health crisis and scared, and I wasn't getting very much of it.

A DIAGNOSIS, FINALLY

The next morning, Friday, I was again the first patient of the day at my neurologist's office — I think because they were fitting me into the schedule.

I sat with my wife in the waiting room, listening to the soothing sounds of a waterfall and the intermittent twang of "environmental" music. Soothing — right. I was ready to stomp the damn CD player into dust.

I was anxious and scared. I was exhausted. But I was also hopeful and excited. I was sure I was about to get some answers. I might not like what I was about to hear, but at least I'd know.

My poor wife was a wreck but had remained a source of strength for me throughout the ordeal. She was clearly ready and determined to hear some answers, too.

The doctor sat us down and wasted no time at all. No pleasantries or small talk, for which I was grateful.

"You have MS — multiple sclerosis," he said. He told me the condition affecting my eye was called optical neuritis (ON) and was one of the top symptoms leading to an MS diagnosis.

Not everyone with optical neuritis has or gets MS, but apparently most do.

He said his diagnosis, based on my MRI and the presence of ON, was pretty much definitive.

I was speechless, and so was my wife, but not for the reasons you may think. I was to learn later that my wife and I had very different takes on what this diagnosis meant.

You see, I had heard whispers in the hospitals and doctors' offices that perhaps I had brain cancer, or a brain tumor. We had heard mention of eye cancer, too. But not once had anyone mentioned MS.

Quite frankly, I was relieved.

I didn't know much about MS. I did associate it with being in a wheelchair, but I thought it couldn't be nearly as bad as some of the other diagnoses I had been worrying about.

My wife, on the other hand was horrified. She knew, far more intimately than I realized or recognized, what an MS "sentence" might mean.

In addition, the blood tests revealed that my cholesterol had gone up, a problem I have had forever. I was told I needed to go back on Lipitor. I had read some scary stuff about the cholesterol-lowering drugs (statins) when researching my wife's cancer and had stopped taking this drug a year earlier. Although my cholesterol was high, it was only marginally high by statistical standards (my statistical standards, but apparently not the doctors').

I was to go home and educate myself regarding the approved MS drugs. Once I had read a pile of stuff from the neurologist and watched some videos he had also given me, I was to make an appointment at the MS clinic. My neuro served as part of the staff there. I was told I would need to choose "quickly" which of the four main MS drugs (often referred to as CRAB drugs — Copaxone, Rebif, Avonex, and Betaserone) I'd like to begin self-injecting. It would be best to start injecting one of these drugs within the next 30 days, I was told, and the clinic would help me with any questions.

Now, you may be asking yourself why the doctor wasn't telling me which drug to take; I certainly was asking myself that question. The best I can figure is that there are two big issues here.

The first is cost. The range in price of these drugs was from more than $1000 a month to well over $2000 a month. I am guessing most doctors don't want to tell their patients they need to take a drug for the rest of their lives they likely can't afford.

The second is that all the CRAB drugs apparently promise about the same level of average effectiveness, but they don't all work equally well on everyone. In fact many MSers end up trying some or all of them during the course of their treatments. So I'm also guessing, given the extreme pressures to choose one so quickly, doctors don't want to be accused of having picked the wrong drug initially.

I had an appointment scheduled with my family doctor for Monday anyway, and he would be sending me for additional blood tests. I was told he would be prescribing Lipitor or a similar drug.

My medical problem had finally been diagnosed, and it seemed the good news was there were medicines to fix it, or at least control it. I had the weekend to wade through all the CRAB-related information.

I had asked about other treatments and medications but was assured by my neurologist the CRAB drugs were my only real choices.

He told me they were the standard of care. (Remember that phrase: "standard of care.")

I guess you could say one benefit of the diagnostic muddle I had been through, and the time it took, was the relief I felt when I finally got my diagnosis. Imagine that — I felt relieved to know I had MS. For about three days.

TWO

MOVING FROM PASSIVITY TO ACTION

Know thy enemy and know thyself and
you will win a hundred battles.
— GENERAL SUN TZU WU

I WENT THROUGH several waves of reaction when I heard my scary diagnosis. At first, as just mentioned, I felt relieved. At least I knew what I was dealing with. But that feeling quickly morphed into numbness.

Looking back, I realize I was in shock. "Shock" is one of those words that get used so often, it has pretty much lost its meaning. I now knew exactly what it meant. I was relieved I didn't have something worse but scared and confused about what was going to happen to me. And so, initially, I shut down. I didn't want to know any more than I had to. My wife recognized this as a problem because normally I am very curious and proactive. Her experiences with her own scary diagnosis of cancer (twice) caused warning bells about my behavior to go off in her head.

She had never seen me frozen like the proverbial deer caught in the headlights, and was sure that nudging me along was going to be a good thing for me in the long run.

As a result of her gentle prodding, I went, in a matter of days, from not wanting to know anything much about MS (most likely as a result of denial) to wanting to know everything there was to know. Once I started, I couldn't stop. I quickly realized not only that little was known about what I was told I had, but also that many differing opinions regarding the "facts" were being presented to me.

A CRAB HUNT

I spent the weekend reviewing the information supplied by my neurologist — expensive glossy brochures and professional DVDS informing me all about MS and the pros and cons of each of the CRAB drugs. Even though I am very comfortable on a computer and Internet savvy, I stayed off the Internet because I was afraid of what I might see and read. I had scared myself big time that way when my wife had her second bout of cancer, malignant melanoma. Some of the stories and pictures I came across were terrifying. Although they clearly were valid stories, many were extreme cases.

I trusted that all I needed to know could be found in the impressive information kits from the doctor. Actually, they were, for the most part, really from the various pharmaceutical companies producing these drugs, and they were state-of-the-art marketing pieces.

As is often the case, the potential side effects of the drugs were almost as scary as the possible effects of the disease itself.

And the *prices* of these drugs — mind-boggling!

The idea of self-injecting was another obstacle.

But the biggest shock was the reported effectiveness of the CRAB drugs. Even the glossy brochures couldn't hide how marginal the potential benefits of these drugs were. It appeared I could only expect about a 30% reduction in MS attacks by taking the drugs — assuming I had the relapsing and remitting kind of MS (often referred to as RRMS); I had been told only time would tell which kind I had.

There are two main ways to categorize cases of multiple sclerosis. Simply put, you can have the kind that attacks and subsides, or you can be under attack constantly, with no time to recover (this type of MS is considered "progressive"). There are additional categories, because some patients are thought to be somewhere between these two.

Furthermore, it seemed one's body could begin to reject these drugs over time or they could just stop working (assuming they were working to begin with). Having been told I had no viable options other than the CRAB drugs, I began to squirm a bit. Actually, I could barely sit still.

Be that as it may (I couldn't resist just one more time), I made up my mind to be the perfect patient and report to the MS clinic as soon as possible. I'd ask the list of questions I had accumulated from my weekend studies, and begin injecting myself within the next two weeks.

I could tell my wife wasn't comfortable with this, but she didn't say anything — yet. I, like most folks, was concerned about whether I could even stick a needle into myself. These drugs require intramuscular injections, which means putting a big needle deep into the muscle.

The actors on the DVDs assured me it was no big deal.

I'm sure it wasn't, for them.

The seeds of doubt about this entire course of action were beginning to sprout.

THE CLINIC

Wednesday, February 25, was my first and last visit, to date, to the MS clinic.

The clinic was a busy place. The reading material was mostly medical and the CRAB drugs were well represented. My wife and I were called into a small conference room and a representative of the clinic began to give me an overview of what they did and how they could help me.

The literature placed in front of us made a large and impressive pile. It appeared to have been carefully arranged to fit the order of the verbal presentation. It made sense that this was a well-rehearsed process, given that it's a regular part of educating a new patient.

To our surprise, the presentation began with the statement it was likely I would need some kind of walking aid in the next seven to ten years, particularly if I did not choose a CRAB therapy.

I was asked to open the top pamphlet, which talked about wheelchairs, with related suggestions and resources to help finance said wheelchair. Next was a pamphlet about the cost of the CRAB therapies and how there are few if any government programs or insurance companies that help pay for the treatments (at least, few that would help pay long-term, and the sense of the material was that I would need to be on them forever).

The presentation went on like this for quite a while, but I pretty much stopped listening at the part about the wheelchair. My legs were basically fine, so did I really need to hear this? Besides, the presentation was sounding more and more like an infomercial for the CRAB drugs and the companies that made them.

The sun was quickly setting on my hopes that any talk about a cure would materialize.

One thing that put me off the idea of sticking with the clinic was that it was located in the same university-affiliated hospital I had been to at the start of all this. The clinic was in the same complex as the ER I had turned to twice initially — in fact, it was practically next door to it. I was now being told I had "classic" MS symptoms, and that, based on those symptoms, any medical student could have figured out what was wrong with me almost immediately.

Unfortunately for me, I had seen just about everyone *but* a medical student.

I told the clinic representatives about my ER visits and asked how it could be that the hospital's own ER doctors hadn't even considered MS as a diagnosis when the clinic was less than a stone's throw from the ER. "We don't really know," was the answer.

There seemed way too much no one knew, and I wasn't convinced they even knew what they said they knew.

WHY I DIDN'T GO BACK

It may sound as if I'm ungrateful for the resources available to MS patients or for the existence of MS clinics (or the other specialty clinics available for almost any serious health problem), but that couldn't be further from the truth. I have tremendous respect for all those doctors, nurses, and other folks who work or volunteer at any clinic or association or society. They mean well and are essential for some of the victims of these potentially terrible conditions or diseases. Most of them do some amazing work for those who need help the most, and they may be a last hope for those least able to cope financially or physically. This clinic seemed directly related to the local branch of the MS Society. (There are many somewhat independent MS societies worldwide. At the time I thought they were all under one administration and management.)

I appreciated the opportunity to attend the clinic, and I hope their good works continue. I would like to see some refocusing of their priorities, but that's for another time.

But this approach was simply not for me and may not be for you. These groups may even have a downside, limiting the options you're willing to consider for moving forward (by omitting or censoring information), or simply having a discouraging or depressing effect on you.

As for specific reasons why the clinic wasn't for me, the first was that not much help was available for my symptoms. Once you receive a diagnosis like MS or are labeled with any other autoimmune issue, you and the doctors will often look back and blame that condition for all sorts of undiagnosed stuff from your past. This happens with many scary diagnoses. Some things probably were the result of whatever you are now labeled with (assuming that the label is correct), and some probably weren't, but the book is now closed on all of them (often prematurely).

In my case those earlier symptoms included some problems I had experienced several years back: a numb and stiff right side (occasionally referred to as partial paralysis, an MS hug, etc.) and a numb left arm and hand. At one point I lost the use of the pinkie on my left hand for a while.

My arm, hand, and finger had more or less gotten better, at least to the point where I didn't notice the weakness. My left leg felt odd, but that may or may not have been because of MS. MS often does affect the legs, but apparently the conventional wisdom was that nothing could be done about it anyway, and if MS was not the cause of the problem, then it wasn't important to the clinic.

Another reason the clinic wasn't for me had to do with the pile of information they had waiting for me, along with some of the statistics they wanted to discuss. Being an engineer by education and by nature, I know all too well how statistics can be used and abused. A "statistical artist" can use them to paint almost any picture desired.

According to the statistics, the high-risk age for MS was 20 to 40, and two-thirds of MS victims were women.

So far this didn't describe me at all.

The number of people believed to have MS was then presented. (I have intentionally omitted the number here because of what I think MS really is and how understated this statistic is; stay tuned for more on that.) I was also told MS doesn't cause death (apparently not exactly true, but death as a result or side effect of the disease is rare). Next came disclaimers about how the CRAB drugs only cut down "attacks" by 30% and don't stop progression. Only 30% — yikes!

ENTER — AND EXIT — MY CLINIC TEAM

The third reason had to do with a so-called team that would be assisting me. I was told I would have a team of professionals at my disposal. It would include staff neurologists, a psychologist, a physiotherapist, a trained nurse, and a coordinator.

I asked about a nutritionist because I thought (and have since come to truly believe) that any health issue has a nutritional component. I began leaning this way during my wife's cancers.

No, nutrition was not considered important and no nutritionist was available.

I said I would see the psychologist, which would be my first-ever such session. Talking about how I was feeling seemed like it might be helpful and perhaps make things easier on my wife. Unfortunately, that person was on maternity leave or had otherwise left (I don't recall which) and had not been replaced. So, no psychologist for me.

Thankfully, I didn't require physical therapy. If I had, I would have been in for a long wait. That position had been vacated (or maybe this was the maternity leave — I just can't remember anymore) and was not yet filled.

The program was clearly a lot better on paper than in practice.

All the information I was getting and some of what I had read was setting off some alarm bells.

I was rapidly discovering that even what was being presented as fact was not. It was a best guess at best.

TAKING CHARGE

I did come to know one thing for sure: It was time for me to wake up and take charge.

I was beginning to feel essentially on my own as far as getting the best possible results for my future. Things didn't look particularly good, nor did it appear, based on what I now thought about the clinic and the CRAB drugs, that I had a solid base to work from.

However, I had always been self-sufficient and knew I needed at least to start trying to figure this out.

I was ready to stand and fight. It was time to wage war. That may sound a bit dramatic, but it was true. It's why I quoted, "Know thy enemy and know thyself and you will win a hundred battles" by General Sun Tzu Wu to begin this chapter. The doctors told me I had been attacked with the first of what were likely to be many attacks. They had also told me my weapons (CRABS) were barely up to the challenge. I was outgunned big time. I needed to know about any and all options. I needed to know my MS enemy and I certainly needed to rely more on myself, my common sense, and my gut instincts if I was going to improve my chances of a better outcome than I'd been shown thus far.

MS is a degenerative condition, which means that even if you get better from its "attacks," you typically don't recover 100%. It eats away at you, giving back less than it takes each time.

I needed several plans for dealing with best- to worst-case scenarios, as no one was sure how severe my case was. This meant my information must be complete, not just the one-sided stuff I'd seen so far. I wanted and needed to see any and all information, whether valid or relevant in someone else's opinion or not.

This was about my body and my life. Who better than I to judge what was and was not important?

I started thinking about the "trust but verify" concept, and what it really meant. The phrase is a quote from Ronald Reagan when he was president of the U.S. He had used it regarding his country's relationship with the Soviets. I started my search for more answers with a big question written on a clean sheet of lined paper: "What is really known about MS — the facts, not the guesses?" As I researched that very first question, I was shocked by where it was leading me.

The second, inevitable question was a bombshell in itself: "Is there really such a thing, a single identifiable disease, as MS? Or is it a general label, a sort of catch-all for folks with some similar symptoms?"

And then I couldn't help but wonder if MS was really a disease at all. Is it a disease one catches, or a condition one develops? And how the heck did I catch or develop it?

Did I really have MS, or did I have one of the many other possible diseases or conditions that could look similar? Many of these had never been mentioned to me in the course of my diagnosis, nor had I even heard of some of them.

All of a sudden I had lots of questions and some serious doubts. I had gone through so much and waited so long, and here I was questioning the doctors and my very own scary diagnosis. How dare I? How could I? The doctors were the experts and I was certainly no doctor.

My doubts were not only about what I was told regarding what I was supposed to have, but also about what I really "had" to begin with. Was my diagnosis even right?

HOW YOU CAN TAKE ACTION

Let me take a break from telling my story to address you and your situation — or the situation of one of your loved ones — more directly.

You may feel your diagnosis doesn't have the margin of error that I'm suggesting mine had and has.

You may think as you read this bit that these kinds of questions don't apply to you.

You may think I was just a bit paranoid or even outright delusional, perhaps as a result of my experiences or symptoms. Maybe he's still in shock, you may be thinking.

Believe it or not, you'd probably be wrong.

In many ways you probably are me, at least with respect to the nature of your condition and diagnosis regardless of what you've been labeled with.

You need to recognize and accept that your first step should be to gather as much relevant information as possible before making any judgments or coming to any conclusions. Look for information that helps you understand and deal with whatever health crisis you're facing. Throughout this book we'll talk a lot about information — how to find it, how to use it, how it gets abused, and how it can trick you. Today, information is more readily available in more ways than ever before. There are books, magazines, talk shows, news shows, specialty channels, clubs, the Internet in general and user groups and forums more specifically — the list goes on and on.

The goal, your goal, is to make your own plan and then implement it. In order to make one with the best chance of working, of helping you, you need information. In order to implement your plan, you'll need a team of people — your team, one you put together. That team includes your doctors, nurses, healthcare providers (often including so-called alternative practitioners), family, friends, and anyone you may need to help you get things moving in the right direction. That team needs a leader, and since this is about you (initially, it should be all about you) and this is happening to you, that leader should be you.

Plans change. A scary diagnosis means change. The more you learn and the more new things get discovered and tried, the more your plans may change. That's a good thing. It's what you want, because the more options you have and try, the better the chances you have to improve your health and life. Embrace change, even though that's very tough for most of us to accept. Once you "got sick," ignoring or resisting change was no longer an acceptable option for you.

AM I DESCRIBING YOU HERE?

I quickly came to the conclusion that no one really knows for sure what MS is or how one gets it. I read several theories about its root causes, suggestions it was genetic, guesses it might be environmental. This seems to be true for most if not all the so-called autoimmune diseases and perhaps many if not most other scary diagnoses. I'd include in that observation most heart and circulation-related stuff and even most cancers. You can be your own judge of this as you begin your own homework.

My wife knew all she had to do was get me started. It may take you a bit more time or effort to become consumed by research and reading, but once you are, you'll find there won't be enough hours in the day to wade through all the stuff you'll come across.

The rest of this book deals with how you can educate yourself about your disease or condition and how to handle your situation psychologically, but let me give you a preview here.

Don't get scared or bogged down with some of the horrible cases and case studies you may come across in books or on the Internet. Many are worst-case scenarios. Many are cases that happened years ago, or that went undiagnosed or untreated. Some were just ignored. Just because "their" case was bad doesn't mean yours needs to be or will be. Always assume you have a mild case of whatever you've been told you've got.

Once you begin to understand what your illness or condition is all about, and any theories or facts about what may have caused it, you'll next want to understand what went into your diagnosis. How definitive was the testing that was done? Are there other things that look a lot like or exactly like what you've been told you have with respect to your symptoms and test results?

Once you get some idea of what has actually happened to you and what has been done to define it, the next thing you want is confirmation. Acquiring and digesting all this information, all this knowledge, takes action. You don't need to become an M.D. overnight. You can get a general feel for what's going on by reading summaries of medical or research papers, and stories of others facing the same kinds of issues you are. You need to learn just enough at first to come up with an initial list of questions. Use your head, draw your own conclusions based on a wide cross-section of information, and listen to your gut.

The trick is getting started. You need to get past the shock and awe. You need to get to work.

This book is based on learning from experience and mistakes, mine and others, so you can hit the ground running and get to the "feeling better" stage faster, rather than spending precious time in the "why me and what do I do now" stage.

You may feel like hiding under the covers and hibernating in bed.

I did, at least at first.

You can probably get away with it for a while just because of your diagnosis and how freaked out you and everyone around you will tend to be.

Actually, it may help if you take the opportunity to hide in bed a bit to digest what you've been told and think about how you're going to proceed. Just don't stay isolated for too long. You may not want to get out of that bed, but often that's really the first step in dealing with your diagnosis and may dictate how you respond to all kinds of issues, both short- and long-term. I'm telling you not to get stuck. It's vitally important for you to snap out of it as soon as possible.

In order to truly get started, you need to pay attention to some basic stuff and face some of the feelings and emotions you may be dealing with. Facing them won't make them disappear but will help you recognize what may be holding you back.

DEALING WITH STRESS

Every scary diagnosis, regardless of what it is, has one thing in common for sure. That thing is stress.

The best way to deal with stress begins with understanding why you're stressed. I know, you're thinking, "He must be kidding — I'm facing the end of life as I know it." But you can change that. You can adapt and move on.

For most of us uncertainty equals stress. The word "stress" is used and abused so much that most people don't take the time (key word) to understand its role in health crises. This is especially true at the beginning of your illness. You need to accept that things have changed and are changing for you, and you need to take care of yourself the best you can. It may be difficult to believe that such changes, some of them no doubt considered "bad" ones, have even the slightest bit of "good" associated with them. Often they do, but it may take some time for you to see what good can possibly result from a life-altering diagnosis.

Exercise and sleep are both important for feeling better and getting better. Both reduce stress and its effects. You should focus on them as a priority regardless of where you are in the process of dealing with your health issues.

Sleep is extra important early in the process. If you can't sleep, especially while you're going through the early stages of an illness and diagnosis, get help. Ask your doctor to prescribe some sleep medication. It may even be covered by your drug or health plan.

I say this even though I am convinced it's extremely critical for people these days to minimize the use of both prescription and over-the-counter drugs. We all seem to take way too many drugs that have far too many unknowns attached to them and side effects to watch for. Remember, these drugs are mixing and interacting with any of the other drugs or chemicals in your body. The number of combinations of interactions can be staggering, well beyond anyone's ability to test or predict with total accuracy.

Of course, always discuss with your pharmacist any potential interactions with your other medication, as you may be taking over-the-counter stuff or getting drugs prescribed by more than one doctor. Be sure to tell every doctor, including any specialist you see, about any and all drugs you may be taking. Never assume they already know or remember *anything*.

As for exercise, for most of us, even the tiniest bit of it is good. Initially, getting out of bed may be all the exercise you can handle. Do a bit of walking — anything just to get your blood flowing and lungs working. As time goes by you can ramp it up a bit. Even if you're in a wheelchair, there are exercises you can do.

You also need to try to do some normal stuff and allow yourself some special treats. Eat your favorite foods (assuming you're allowed to by your doctors), see a movie or DVD, read something entertaining (don't confine your reading to research). Be nice to yourself, at least occasionally.

If you can't stand, get help. Get a cane or a walker or get yourself into a wheelchair and get rolling. Do what you can when you can.

How you respond is what it's all about.

Many people find they can help themselves to get better if they can just get *feeling* a bit better. I realize this could be a chicken-and-egg sort of thing, but I found it true for me. I started to feel better when I started doing something. For the most part, the more research I did and the more I learned — the more stuff I tried — the better I got.

No matter what part you're playing — patient or support person — you will feel better and keep things moving in a positive direction by getting actively involved. Having one person or a group of informed people to discuss things with can be a tremendous help. You can and should play a key role in this ongoing process. Healing takes place on many levels, and being an "educated consumer," whether you're the patient or "other," is the best first step.

THREE

NAVIGATING THE DIAGNOSTIC PROCESS

All truth passes through three stages. First, it is ridiculed.
Second, it is violently opposed.
Third, it is accepted as being self-evident.
— ARTHUR SCHOPENHAUER

WHEN WE GET sick, I mean really sick, the kind of "sick" that results in a scary diagnosis, we start out desperately wanting to know exactly what caused it. We want to know precisely, and in no uncertain terms, why we got sick and how to fix it.

Perhaps this has happened or will happen to you. Perhaps there is a definitive test for what you've got and a simple, effective, clear-cut treatment or even a cure. But in many if not most cases, at least at first, it's a guessing game. Your diagnosis may take some time and may change from day to day and from doctor to doctor.

That was the case for me. Did I really have, for an absolute fact, what they were saying I had? Did I really have MS, a degenerative and incurable disease?

How could I know for sure?

The doctors told me I had MS, and yet the tests never seemed definitive. It took a combination of tests and symptoms to diagnose me, and even then it was noted that I didn't fit the age or gender profile. Although I had some symptoms that presented as "classic," I had others that didn't.

FACT VERSUS FICTION

If I was going to move forward, I needed to separate fact from fiction. I needed to know the whole truth, not just the stuff the doctors wanted to tell me or felt comfortable telling me. Not just what was presented in the shiny drug company pamphlets. And certainly not what a bunch of actors on a DVD were promoting.

I asked myself some tough questions:

— How definitive are these tests?
— Are there any other conditions or diseases with symptoms similar to MS?
— If so, are there tests that can tell whether or not I have one of those "other" things? Have I been given those tests? And how "conclusive" or "inconclusive" are they?
— Are the doctors going to tell me everything — and I mean everything — or do I need some other way to find the complete picture, including all the issues and options?

I realized I needed information. I needed to make lists of questions. Some of those needed to be simple "yes or no" questions. No doctorspeak, no medical jargon or hedging out of fear of being sued down the road; just plain everyday English.

It was as if a switch in my brain had been thrown into the ON position.

THE SEARCH WAS ON

I started thinking, which wasn't easy with my head buzzing. But finally all the lights were on and someone was actually home. I was home. I was back. Well, sort of, anyway.

I was back just enough to ask some of the "right" questions. Now that I knew I had to take control of this, I needed to figure out what to ask and how best to ask it. This was something I was used to doing. One thing about being an engineer, you know how to study something to death, and I do mean grind it right into the ground.

I knew how to review reports and statistics. I knew it was important for me to draw my own conclusions because I also knew that, taken out of context, almost any position based on the "available" information could be justified by someone clever enough.

I decided I was going to be my own judge and jury. I'd look at *all* the information and decide on a plan of action that made sense to *me*. It was time to stop playing defense with my MS diagnosis and start playing offense.

And if that meant being perceived as "offensive" by some of the professionals I was seeing, because I wasn't allowing myself to be led along submissively, so be it.

It's often said "the best defense is a good offense." That certainly applies to health and wellness.

I wished I didn't have to do all this. I wasn't feeling great, and both reading and thinking hurt, but it was my life and I damn well wasn't ready to accept what the MS clinic and some of the doctors were preparing me for at the age of 50. That wasn't even remotely what I had in mind.

I started searching. I scanned books and scoured the Internet.

My list of possible diagnoses now included Lyme disease, mercury toxicity, lupus, vitamin B_{12} deficiency, and others. There were actually different lists, on different Internet sites, of potential conditions or diseases that could look like MS. There was also plenty of disagreement regarding which were valid and which were not. The excerpt below taken from the National Institute of Neurological Disorders and Strokes website is just one example:

> A number of other diseases may produce symptoms similar to those seen in MS. Other conditions with an intermittent course and MS-like lesions of the brain's white matter include polyarteritis, lupus erythematosus, syringomyelia, tropical spastic paraparesis, some cancers, and certain tumors that compress the brainstem or spinal cord. Progressive multi-focal leukoencephalopathy can mimic the acute stage of an MS attack. Physicians will also need to rule out stroke, neurosyphilis, spinocerebellar ataxias, pernicious anemia, diabetes, Sjogren's disease, and vitamin B_{12} deficiency. Acute *transverse myelitis* may signal the first attack of MS, or it may indicate other problems such as infection with the Epstein-Barr or herpes simplex B viruses. Recent reports suggest that the neurological problems associated with Lyme disease may present a clinical picture much like MS.[1]

I'm not saying I thought some of the conditions on such lists would be an improvement on my MS diagnosis. I just wanted, if possible, to at least eliminate these other things.

What if I actually had something that could be easily treated or even cured?

---

1   http://www.ninds.nih.gov/disorders/multiple_sclerosis/detail_multiple_
    sclerosis.htm

Remember, I'm not trying to convince you that your diagnosis is right or wrong. I am urging you to educate yourself and do your best to verify the accuracy of it.

Mercury toxicity popped up at a very regular rate as causing MS-like symptoms. (This topic is covered in greater detail in chapter ten.)

The toxicity of mercury, especially dental mercury, is a major can of worms in and of itself. There are tons of studies and articles saying mercury (in some fish we eat, for example), and particularly mercury from dental fillings (amalgams) and in the air we breathe, may have negative effects on health. But they are argued to be inconclusive and often "unpopular" at best.

There are other articles and studies screaming about mercury-related health issues.

As reported in a Reuters article, scientists from the United Nations Environmental Program (UNEP) concluded in 2002 that mercury was a very serious global issue. "The heavy metal, used in or released by many industrial processes as well as in dentistry and medical thermometers, is transformed by contact with water into a poisonous compound easily absorbed by humans, animals, and fish."[2]

Scary, right?

After reading all I could, I decided this was a viable issue for me and should be included on my list of possible causes of my problems.

Please take this as an example for you and your list. Put yourself in the position where you decide what needs to be included and why.

What's important at this point is the fact I was no longer convinced — and apparently for good reasons — that my scary diagnosis was necessarily accurate.

2   http://www.cbsnews.com/stories/2002/09/13/tech/main522011.shtml

When my symptoms started, I was desperate for a diagnosis, almost any diagnosis. Now that I had one, I was becoming less certain about it every day.

I had crossed the border from the country of denial into the country of doubt.

Some of the other possible conditions did have potential treatments, ones that seemed more likely to get and keep me stable and healthy. What if my symptoms were simply the result of a Vitamin B_{12} deficiency, for example?

If I had the wrong diagnosis, how could I hope to apply the appropriate treatments?

SCRUTINIZE YOUR CONDITION

Take another hard look at what they say you have. I did.

I found out no one knows what causes MS. In fact there are at least three or four viable theories, none of which can be proved or disproved.

Until recently MS was primarily considered an autoimmune disease — a disease that, in simple terms, resulted from your body attacking itself via your immune system. In MS, your immune system is thought to be attacking the myelin covering your nerves, apparently for no obvious reason. You can think of your nerves as wires and myelin as the insulation on those wires; if the insulation gets damaged, the wire can short out. It has been theorized recently that the myelin gets sick or begins to die. Again, the reason is unclear, but according to this theory that's why your immune system kicks in. In this theory, it is not attacking all of the myelin and for no reason. Rather, it's attacking myelin that is getting sick or dying in order to get it out of the system.

The difference may be huge when it comes to discovering the actual cause and potential treatments or cures.

Others believe a viral connection causes or triggers MS.

Still others believe it's triggered by bacteria, or a fungus, or even a parasite. In keeping with the bacteria theory, some trials are focusing on using antibiotics (like minocycline) to treat MS, as opposed to the standard of care that encourages injection of one of the CRAB drugs thought to suppress or otherwise moderate the immune system. A recent study questions whether this kind of suppression or moderation increases the MS patient's chances of being stricken with cancer (as if we don't have enough to worry about). Some of the MSers being treated with minocycline (the antibiotic) are reporting impressive results, which would support a bacterial connection, while others apparently are not.

Accepting a new theory as to why MS happens would probably result in reclassification of the disease as something other than an autoimmune disease. When will it be possible, if ever, to "prove" whether any of the theories is 100% correct? No telling.

It's interesting to note that the CRAB drugs and other standard-of-care regimes are based on the autoimmune theory. If that theory proves to be incorrect, what would that say about these treatments?

One thing almost everyone agrees with is that no two MS patients have exactly the same combination of symptoms, or experience the disease, if it is a disease, in the same way.

Here's a list of possible symptoms of multiple sclerosis. There are many lists that may differ slightly depending on who put each list together and when.

- Muscle weakness
- Spasticity

- Impairment of pain, temperature, touch senses
- Pain (moderate to severe)
- Ataxia
- Tremor
- Speech disturbances
- Vision disturbances
- Vertigo
- Bladder dysfunction
- Bowel dysfunction
- Sexual dysfunction
- Depression
- Euphoria
- Cognitive abnormalities
- Fatigue[3]

As you can see, MS can look and feel like many things. Similar lists can be compiled for all kinds of illnesses. This is especially true of the so-called autoimmune diseases.

Clearly, I had my work cut out for me, though it seemed to me that finding out what was wrong with me could well turn out to be an unattainable goal.

So, what to do?

I decided to deal with the things I could control, or at least influence. My doctors and the MS clinic said diet wasn't an issue. They said mercury wasn't an issue. They also said Lyme disease (sometimes described as an arthritic-like condition mainly affecting the large joints, caused by a bacteria transmitted by ticks and possibly other biting insects or through the exchange

---

3   http://www.ninds.nih.gov/disorders/multiple_sclerosis/detail_multiple_
    sclerosis.htm

of bodily fluids) was rare in Canada and not a priority.

They had said lots of stuff that common sense prompted me to question.

WHAT IS A DIAGNOSIS?

In fact, starting at the beginning, what does the word "diagnosis" mean, anyway? Here's how the *Cambridge Advanced Learner's Dictionary* defines it:

diagnosis
noun [C or U] plural diagnoses
a judgment about what a particular illness or problem is, made after making an examination:

"What was the diagnosis?" "Arthritis in both joints."
The doctor has made an initial diagnosis, but there'll be an additional examination by a specialist.
Diagnosis of the disease (= saying what it is) is difficult in the early stages.[4]

Notice it says a "judgment." A diagnosis doesn't say this is what you've got for sure. It's clearly just a best guess.

The last example in the definition reads: "Diagnosis of the disease (= saying what it is) is difficult in the early stages." That may be an understatement.

Doesn't that get you thinking about doctors and medicine? Is medicine a science or an art, or some combination of the two?

Let's remember something. Regardless of what your preconceived

---

4   http://dictionary.cambridge.org/define.asp?key=21449&dict=CALD

notions are or were of doctors and modern medicine, doctors are people. They may be well educated and highly trained and have lots of experience, but they are people.

Just like any of us, they can and do make mistakes, and more often than you may think. They don't have all the answers. I started to see the "practice" of medicine as just that. Modern medicine is part art and part science. The doctors are practicing and learning in an effort to get better at it, to figure it out. What is often presented as medical fact today may well be proven medical fiction tomorrow. A wonder drug today may be banned tomorrow (sound familiar?).

I decided to change my mental picture of doctors and medicine. I decided to change my expectations. Some folks would use the phrase "I changed my paradigm." I had to. I realized I had unreal expectations. I'm guessing this may also be true of you.

Believe me, I respect and appreciate doctors. It's a job I would not want to do myself. But now I recognize they are not the old-time television-style personalities I had grown up with. In fact, I believe the more recent television medical dramas are more realistic regarding what actually happens day to day. Ever see *House, M.D.?* The guys on that program get the diagnosis wrong several times, in every case, every time, before getting it right.

But for most folks, these newer television shows are just entertainment. They require little thought and have little effect on how they perceive the medical world. At least when it comes to them and their families, people don't want to believe medicine is chaotic and diagnosis is typically a guessing game . They want to believe all doctors know it all — that they will, without a doubt, figure out what's wrong with them and how to fix it.

It's frustrating but ultimately liberating to realize that, for the most part, what doctors are really trying to do is guess correctly as often as possible. The good ones guess right more often than they guess wrong.

It's up to you to help shift the odds of guessing right in your favor.

When you initially hear your scary diagnosis, the first thing you need to do is confirm, the best you can, whether it's correct.

Many first-time diagnoses are at least partially correct, but far too many are wrong and so deserve serious scrutiny — your scrutiny. I've read that between 40% and 60% of patients who have received a diagnosis believe they initially received an incorrect one.

The truth is, many conditions today do not have definitive tests, and their diagnosis relies heavily on your symptoms and your doctors' observations. That means they're guessing.

MY OPINION ON MEDICAL OPINIONS

You need a second, third, or numerous additional "opinions" if you're ever going to get "comfortable" with what you've been told you have.

However, new "opinions" should be based on *new* tests. Test results change and can be wrong. Your doctors or insurance companies may try to block you when you set out to undergo further scrutiny, but you need to insist on new tests, new pictures, and start-from-scratch examinations. Do not let anyone assume anything or get lazy.

In my opinion, second opinions based on original test data are often a waste of time. They can lead to automatic confirmation of the initial diagnosis, or occasionally result in a contradictory diagnosis that requires additional testing anyway.

Here is a great example of what I'm talking about. An MRI of my brain was part of my diagnostic process, and although I could see the pictures on a computer screen, they needed to be read by a radiologist. The radiologist's report was sent to my neurologist (the doctor who diagnosed me). That report said it was fairly definitive that I had MS.

I sent a copy of that very same MRI, without the written report, to a relative who's a radiologist. He had two other neuroradiologists read it, and their report contradicted the first one. It concluded that if the "patient" (meaning me) was not symptomatic, the MRI was basically normal for a 50-year-old male. Yet, if they were to examine me, they would realize something major was wrong. In this example, I didn't need another MRI, I needed a fresh interpretation of the original one. The MRI itself was just a picture and was fine.

Clearly there's a lot of room for error. It's fine to get a second opinion using the original tests, but only if new tests are done as well.

We could debate whether it's better to start from scratch by telling the new doctor everything or nothing of what you already know about the first diagnosis. That choice is best made on an individual basis, because it needs to take several factors into account.

These factors include looking at the statistical reliability of the test(s) associated with your diagnosis. Were all the tests available done at least once? Does your diagnosis require observation as a primary means of identifying your illness, and testing as secondary? Are your symptoms "classic," or are there symptoms that seem related but don't fit the general profile of your diagnosis? Once you take a hard look at all the available information about reaching a diagnosis for your illness and compare it with what has been done diagnostically to you so far, it should be relatively simple to make a list of possible tests and questions that are specific to you.

Once you're reasonably certain you and your team (doctors, professional practitioners, family, etc.) know what you really have, you should focus on what you can do about it.

It is important to repeat here once again that many diseases and conditions don't have any definitive tests. This means the tests that are performed don't say you *absolutely* have or don't have a particular disease or condition. Many look for indicators or co-factors.

In other words, you may never know what you have for sure. What you're hearing is often a best guess. At some point you will need to decide whether to make do with that guess. That decision point is different for each of us, and reaching it becomes part of the process I'm describing here.

Even if definitive tests do exist for what you've got, that doesn't mean anybody really knows with any degree of certainty what *causes* the illness you tested positive for. Not knowing the cause leaves room for error when deciding on treatments.

Don't believe me? Check it out yourself with a quick Internet search. See if anyone really knows exactly how and why you got what you got.

In the end, confirming your diagnosis often becomes about eliminating any and all of the "other" things you may have, based on your symptoms. It's often up to you to make sure this process of elimination actually happens.

FOUR

NAVIGATING PERSONAL ISSUES

The physician should not treat the disease
but the patient who is suffering from it.
— MAIMONIDES

D-DAY.

For us patients that means Diagnosis Day.

It's the day the old you, the person you were your whole life, disappears and a new, frailer, mortal you appears.

That's what happened to me, and I believe it's what happens to most people after being diagnosed with something serious. The day you tell someone your diagnosis is the day their mental picture of you changes forever. I can typically tell how other people feel about me now based on their questions and concerns. They actually "look" at me differently, even though any limitations resulting from my condition, so far, aren't obvious.

The conditions and symptoms that led to your scary diagnosis are life-changing. But often they don't have to be as draining as you initially thought. You almost always have some choices, and making the right ones is part of taking control of and responsibility for your wellness. You may not be able to choose whom to tell about your diagnosis if your symptoms are obvious. But you may have that choice with friends or loved ones who live far from you. How you tell them will depend on what works best for you. You need to be in control because this is first of all about you. At the beginning, anyway, they aren't even a close second.

In many ways I consider myself to be a completely different person since my diagnosis. Not just a new me, but a new person. How others who know about my condition see me has certainly changed, but the biggest and most important change is how I see myself.

TELLING FAMILY

It was almost two and a half years after my diagnosis that I told my parents about receiving an MS diagnosis. (They also didn't know about my eye or the earlier symptoms affecting my side, arm, and leg.) I struggled long and hard with the decision not to tell them. I concluded there was nothing they could do to help and realized I could continue to hide it from them because I lived so far away.

I just didn't want them to focus on my condition. I didn't want to see "that look" in their eyes every time we visited. I wanted us all to focus on our relationships and on the quality of the time we were spending together.

Besides, my mother and stepfather are both around 80 and have their own health issues to deal with.

My wife and I usually visit my family two or three times a year, and I had to cancel only one trip and delay another to hide my diagnosis from them. Sometimes I felt bad about not telling them, or even sorry for myself, but these feelings evaporated every time I saw their faces when we visited, and every Monday when I phoned my mother to chat.

A VOW OF SILENCE

I am not telling you to be a martyr or to suffer alone. You don't need or want to be alone too much, and you certainly shouldn't be silent. My wife's support and patience were, and are, beyond description. She and I talk regularly about what I'm experiencing.

Putting your true feelings and experiences into words in a constructive fashion can be very helpful. This is a good stress-relief tip. Keeping too much "inside" often results in those feelings "eating" their way out. Although I typically picture "eating" as a good thing, in this case it's unequivocally bad.

I told my sisters early on, swearing them to secrecy. I kind of had to tell them because one of them is married to a radiologist, and, as described in the previous chapter, I wanted his opinion on several issues. I also reasoned that I would be really angry if they hid something like this from me. They are young enough, and focused enough on their own lives and families, to deal with my situation and move on. I am also, for the most part, candid about updating them on how things are going when I'm asked.

Sometimes I think the "universe" steps in to smooth things over or to set things right. Here's an example.

After finishing the first draft of this book, I was visiting my family and decided to ask my stepfather to read it. By this time he knew about my diagnosis. We had been in Florida together the year before and I had been injecting B_{12} daily at the time. He had found the bag with the vial and needles stuffed in the back of the fridge. What he was doing bent down exploring the depths of the back of the bottom shelf of the refrigerator remains a mystery to me. But then again, what I was doing with all this stuff was a mystery to him. I had to reveal my diagnosis — otherwise he would have thought I was on illegal drugs.

After the visit, my mom found the draft of the book. My stepfather and I had agreed to keep it secret. But within days she found it. Mom rarely goes into the room he reads in, but decided to do so and also decided to turn over the book he'd been reading to see what it was. She saw my name on the manuscript underneath it and began to read it. Next thing I knew, phone calls, faxes, and emails were winging their way to our house, cell phones, and office. If we had a family bat signal the sky would have been ablaze. My sisters were freaking out because my mother had "discovered" the whole truth, and, needless to say, was pretty close to hysterical.

In retrospect, I still think I was right not to have told her initially. But now the timing was probably right. I was uncomfortable hiding it from her, and once she finished reading this book, she not only started to accept what had happened to me but began taking some action of her own. After all, I was two years past "fuzzy eye" and doing pretty well. I looked normal and most of my symptoms weren't visible. There was little reason for her to be upset other than dealing with what the MS label conjured up in her mind.

My mom is more than a decade past a serious bypass operation. She has some other issues and takes a handful of drugs every day. She often complains about how some of the drugs make her feel. As a result of reading my story, she began questioning why she was on so much medication and whether they were working properly together. With the help of my sisters (who also read this book), she had a doctor review her medications (her prescriptions are from several different doctors) and ended up taking fewer medications and in lower doses and dealing proactively with some issues she'd been avoiding.

She also began reading articles and books and watching television shows on health and wellness. We now often discuss some of this stuff in our weekly chats. What started out as a disaster (my mom finding the book) resulted in one of my first satisfied customers (reader of this book). I had wanted to include a "testimonial" from her but I'm guessing one from my mom wouldn't be overly impressive to you.

TELLING OTHERS

As far as non-family connections are concerned, at first I did tell most people I knew locally.

We told the people we worked with, and some of our friends who live close by. I had to, really, because it would have been impossible to hide. For the first three months I was away from the office seeing doctors and undergoing tests. My wife took me to many of these appointments, which could have raised suspicions something was wrong with her.

We have a large circle of business friends — or perhaps acquaintances is a better description — who heard the news through the grapevine, which is certainly faster than any other method of communication known to man.

Quite frankly, I was surprised, hurt, and discouraged by the lack of attention and support, both initially and on an ongoing basis, from some of these people. I'm being brutally honest about this because I don't want you to think, should this happen to you, that it's only happening to you.

Some of my business acquaintances seemed to think I was no longer relevant or otherwise important. These days I choose to believe that they apparently misunderstood what I had told them or what others had told them about what had happened to me. I am guessing that instead of hearing I had been diagnosed with MS, they had received news that I had been dematerialized and sent to Mars. "Diagnosed with MS" and "dematerialized to Mars" sort of sound the same, don't they?

I figure this explains why I never heard from some of them again (or only on the rare occasions when solar flares allow intergalactic communications).

Some people get weird when a disease or illness is mentioned. I used to be one of them. I believe some of these people were picturing themselves in my position, getting stuck on how they would feel if they were me. Part of their reactions had to do more with *their* fears and insecurities than with me.

Preoccupied in this way, they just didn't know how to express themselves in a constructive or helpful fashion. I get that now.

That's why I have forgiven anyone who decided to ignore us or cut loose from my wife and me. Any void left by those who chose to move on has been more than adequately filled by others, thank you very much.

The point is, tell the people *you* feel *you* need to tell.

This is about *you*. This is a time to be "selfish." When it comes to the drama associated with your diagnosis, they are merely observers, whereas you are playing the lead role.

I told one of my oldest friends, Billy, via email, because sometimes you have to tell someone strong and supportive, and I knew he would be. He also lives far away and I knew I wouldn't be seeing him for a while.

An email may sound a bit casual, but often I found it easier to write about what was happening to me rather than discuss it on the phone or face to face. You can control the "conversation" by carefully drafting your words rather than emotionally blurting stuff out. I recommend this method of communication, at least at first. Of course, actually writing and sending a letter would work, too.

I also needed to write things down because I was spending a lot of time on the phone saying the same thing to people seeking help with their own scary diagnosis. The calls got too long and complicated. The interesting thing is that writing was like having a conversation. My emails, and the responses to them, were honest, concise, and to the point. I could also cut and paste pieces of them to customize my messages for different people.

Billy understood the benefits both for the readers of my emails and for me, the writer. He felt the same way when he heard I was writing this book. His reaction, in both cases, makes sense because of who he is as a person and because he writes for (and produces) popular television shows for a living.

Write about what has happened to you and how you feel even if you end up tossing it in the trash, shredding it, or building a sacrificial fire with it. If you do save what you've written, it will also be interesting for you to look back on what you wrote once you're stable and start to normalize.

These days I may or may not answer "I'm fine," if asked. I decided early on, after my diagnosis, to be honest with people about what was happening to me if they asked me. Some seemed to think I was being unnecessarily and brutally honest. People often ask how you're doing but don't really want to know. But why not tell people how I really felt, particularly if I had chosen to tell them about my diagnosis to begin with?

When face to face with people I'd often say something like, "I have been diagnosed with MS. I'm fine with it and you need to be, too. So what's new with you?" Some people laughed out loud (I would, too) because of how in their face I was when I told them. They didn't know how else to react. Others were shocked but moved on. The important thing is that this worked for me. I could say what needed to be said and not get stuck in the awkwardness of the situation. I believe many of those people started out shocked but ended up grateful to me for making my news "easy" on them.

Any cognitive blips that I occasionally have are usually easy for me to cover up. A small joke about stuttering or being unable to think of a word or name, or do simple math, can divert someone's attention from my difficulty. Diverting people's attention from something you don't want them to notice is an old magician's trick, one you may find handy on occasion.

I was the same person I was before my "health crisis," except no one really thought that, including me. So another person I am becoming more honest with is me. Not only about how I feel about me, but also about how I feel about others.

FEELING BETTER, GETTING BETTER

I am getting better at moving on, and accepting and even embracing the changes happening to me almost daily. I think that's one reason why most of my changes have been good rather than "degenerative" (a word commonly used to describe what happens with MS).

Since university I had pictured myself as a disciplined, business-oriented individual, a logical person. I worked hard. Sometimes I made sure others knew it, but often I tried to make it look easy. I did little that was art-related (spontaneous and creative versus intellectual), and excelled at being stiff and aloof.

Spiritually I wasn't sure who or what I was. I can't say that I'm 100% sure now, but I can say that allowing myself to explore my emotional and spiritual sides has thrown open some pretty amazing doors — some that were open just a crack, or not at all, before.

Today I recognize that I was only part of who I can and should be. In some ways these emotional and spiritual deficiencies, which influenced my daily actions, contributed to my illness. I have come to be very sure that this is true. I believe it's a topic that's often ignored and left unexplored in most scary diagnoses.

Recognizing who I was gave me lots of clues to what I needed to work on. I clearly needed to complete myself as part of feeling and getting better.

THE BENEFITS OF DEALING WITH PERSONAL ISSUES

I believe you will see the benefits of the approach I'm advising you to take by looking at who I am today in comparison with my pre-diagnosis self.

I'm a person focused on being as healthy as possible physically and mentally, and growing as much as possible emotionally and spiritually.

I'm trying to really pay attention to what others are saying and feeling and be a positive part of their day. Trust me, before my diagnosis that was not the case.

For me, part of changing is learning about things that are relatively new to me, like health and wellness. It's not only about knowing what to do but actually doing it.

I'm taking all kinds of actions, including teaching myself guitar and writing this book to help others. It's been said that writing is very therapeutic. It has been for me.

I am also working daily on being patient, when appropriate, and being understanding, when necessary, without getting stressed to the point of internal turmoil.

I now recognize I can't afford to waste time on foolishness, and I feel good about having little patience for it.

Perhaps it's a bit of a cliché to say my condition caused an "awakening," but it's true. I believe I "see" others more clearly than ever, even though the sight in my left eye can be an issue. And it's getting easier to accept or reject interaction with people based on what I see, and to feel good about having and making those choices.

GETTING SUPPORT

One way to feel less alone in dealing with your scary diagnosis is to join a user group or forum on the Internet. I'll talk more about the technical details of how to find and join one later, in chapter six, but for now let me just mention the benefits.

When I first started to read posts on many of the user groups I came across, I was shocked.

I was shocked that there was such a fantastic resource available to me.

I was shocked that there were so many other people dealing with many of the same issues and feeling the same way I was, and talking about it to each other.

I was shocked no one had told me about the existence of these groups or forums and particularly about the benefits of interacting with others in similar situations. The ability to compare experiences and learn from what others have gone through is tremendous, and so is the support and hope most groups provide.

User groups are basically online support groups and more. You may choose to join these groups on the Net or prefer to find and attend a group that meets locally — or do both. User groups online generally discuss a much wider range of topics. And they are available 24/7.

Sometimes you need to be able to seek support anonymously just by interacting with others like you, and that's what a user group is good for. But, long-term, you and those close to you will likely be the best support for each other.

YOU AND YOUR LOVED ONES

If you are a loved one reading this, I hope this helps you understand that *you* may go through really big stuff of your own related to a scary diagnosis. You need to decide how to deal with it. You need to figure out what's best for you and the patient. That may look one way in the short term, another way in the long term. My wife decided to be strong, silent, and supportive, short-term. That's what she thought I needed, and she was right. That's what most patients need. Long-term she needed to tell me how she really felt, and as it turns out, I needed to hear it.

I had made some assumptions about how my wife felt about my illness and how she was handling what was happening to me. She's a calm and level-headed person. She survived two bouts of cancer and is fine today. She was a rock. She also, as it turns out, is a great actress. If I could nominate her for an Academy Award, I would. The performance she gave during the first 45 days of my "attack," as she almost dragged me from doctor to doctor, hospital to hospital, and lab to lab, was nothing short of amazing.

She had me fooled. And I don't fool that easy — but hey, I was pretty sick and scared and freaked out, so gimme a break.

I misread her support and calm empathetic concern for me as her being relatively okay with what was happening.

I know what it's like to be the loved one in this situation. The shoe had been on the other foot when I was helping her through her bouts with cancer. Tough as that was, in a way I wasn't totally tuned in to what she was going through — perhaps because I believed she would recover (and she did). For some reason, I never doubted that for a minute. Undoubtedly, I was in shock.

It took me far too long to really get it.

It was two years into my own saga that my wife told me how scared she had really been about my diagnosis. It happened when she read the first draft of this book and realized she needed to set me straight. Her honesty has been very helpful to me. It has also been helpful to us as a couple and family, and I believe made this a better book for most readers.

In fact, here is a statement from this fabulous human being, my wife, Deborah Goodwin Geller, herself:

I honestly don't know which is worse, receiving a scary diagnosis yourself or watching your spouse receive one. Maybe comparing which is worse is a waste of time. Actually, they are different. When you are diagnosed, as terrifying as it can be, your next focus can be on action: What do I do? What can I do? When it's a loved one, you ask the same questions but feel so powerless. You can't do their treatments for them. What can you do?

Taking Alan around to all the doctors he saw before he was diagnosed was nerve-wracking for both of us but I kept positive, hoping for a simple solution. Even though I already knew doctors don't always have the answer, I was hopeful for him.

The day before he received his diagnosis, I had attended the funeral of the mother of a co-worker who had died from complications of her MS. I still had the picture of her in my mind when we went to the doctor. She was bedridden, blind, and couldn't speak. When the doctor told us Alan had MS, I felt my stomach drop. My heart seemed to stop beating. I wanted to scream. I didn't want to upset Alan. He seemed so calm. How could he be? I was so frightened for him.

Truthfully, I was also angry. I felt like we'd had enough. Come on, God, give us a break. MS? You've got to be kidding me. I had pictures of Annette Funicello and Richard Prior running through my mind.

Now, just in case you think I'm a self-centered, spoiled brat, let me just say, I've lost a brother at a young age, and both parents, had two aunts in wheelchairs, and much more I won't go into. (A second brother died tragically this year.) I've never felt like a victim; in fact, quite the opposite. I've always been grateful for my life.

But this was so hard. Alan is not only the love of my life

but, funny as this may sound, *I actually like this guy*. There is no one I respect more. I was heartbroken for him, not for me. I knew I could handle whatever came. Wheelchair? Hospital? I knew I had family help, too, which many people don't. As a matter of fact, my brother, Brad, told me right away, "Don't worry, I'll help you. We know how to deal with people in wheelchairs. We can do this together."

But I also knew Alan had just reached a time in his life when he truly felt free. Free to do what he wanted. Make the choices he wanted. Have a little fun for a change. And now this ... Come on.

You see, I knew I could go through it, but I didn't know if he could. I have a lot of faith. His is growing, but was not the same at that time. I actually had visions he would ask me to "help him die" at some time in the future. I know, for such a positive person, I certainly was thinking of the worst possible scenario.

We drove to the drugstore after leaving the doctor and I was literally in pain trying to control my tears. He still seemed so calm. Of course I realized later he was so relieved he didn't have brain cancer, he thought MS was the good news. When he asked me in the car later, "Do I have what Michael J. Fox has?" I knew he didn't quite realize what he had. As for when he did realize it, boy, was I unaware of what would happen then.

We were supposed to look over the videos the doctor gave us and make a decision within 30 days on what medicine to use. We waited until Sunday to view it. That weekend I would sneak off to the bathroom to cry and then come out and be calm. I'm not saying this is how to handle things, I'm just sharing how I handled it. I kept praying for an answer.

I never said, "Why me?" or Why him?" After all, why not? But I sure was hoping for a miracle. I would wake up in the night, panicked. Again, not for me, but for him. I was mourning his dreams for his future. I was going to be with him all the way, good or bad, but I wasn't sure how he was going to handle this dramatic change in his life.

The other really scary thing for me was seeing the change in him. Alan is a thinker. He is smart, logical, and always ready to do research. I'm sure a lot of you women can relate to this, but whenever it was time to buy some kind of electronics or something for the house, Alan had to shop around and then research all his options on the Internet or in *Consumer Guide* magazine before making the purchase. It can drive me nuts. However, I knew he always made great decisions.

But here he was with a possible life-threatening illness and he was handing himself over to the doctors. This wasn't the guy I knew. Had I lost him already? I have a description of Alan that all our friends know, that "he's like a dog with a bone." He won't let go of something until he masters it, no matter how hard he has to try. Yet here he was, saying, "The doctor said ..." and with seemingly no desire to do his usual research. Was I going to have to mourn the loss of his personality, too?

Back to the video we got from the doctor. We watched, cried a little, and *counted our blessings*. Yes, you got that right. As we saw how expensive the medicine would be, and how much help we might need, we were so grateful that we'd been successful in business and conservative with our money.

At the same time we caught the first glimpse of what was to become a mission for us. We were getting angry for the people who didn't have the same choices we had. What about the mom with four kids who can't afford the medicine? Or the man whose insurance will cover it up to four years? Which four years does he pick?

Then we had to choose which side effects we thought were going to be the easiest to handle. The literature for one drug said, "When you take this you'll feel like you are having a heart attack." The literature for another said, "You'll feel like you have the flu soon after taking this." Of course, both drugs were to be taken regularly.

Yet another said, "You may develop a resistance to this medication." One of the drugs was a form of Interferon, which I had taken for my cancer. I knew the horrible side effects of that drug, including some instances of suicide due to the depression it can cause. I wouldn't wish it on anyone.

Again I waited to see some sign of the Alan I knew. He showed up a few days later. We had gotten into the habit of my going to bed early, followed by him later. He slept late — not unusual when you're getting depressed. Then one morning he said, "I was on the Internet last night ..." I thought, oh God, please let this be it. Let this be the first step in Alan coming back to himself. It didn't matter to me what he found out, just that he was not giving up so easily.

Hope is so valuable in times like these. He also told me he was making a list of questions for our MS clinic appointment. I secretly thought, "Boy, they won't know what hit them when he walks in." He had 29 questions for them by the time we got there.

Of course he tells you that story, but I just wanted to tell you how it felt from my perspective. Alan was there for me when I had both cancer issues. I wanted to be there for him and yet let him handle it the way he wanted. We each handle illness differently, which isn't unusual between men and women. What I knew for sure was we couldn't just give in.

As a matter of fact, when we went back to see the neurologist, I told him, "Listen, we are solution-oriented people, not problem-oriented. We want some options."

I don't want to leave you with any kind of impression that I am anything but normal. I am in no way a superwoman. I had fears, anger, sadness, and even — I hate to say it — some selfishness. I was worried the stress of this could bring my cancer back. Every day was a battlefield of the mind and I had to be ready for that fight. I also had to realize this was now his full-time job, and like any job we'd be talking about it every day.

Every day Alan learned more. I honestly feel like he's done a university degree in this subject. I saw him gain strength physically, mentally, and spiritually. He looks healthier and *is* healthier than he was before his diagnosis. He's also more compassionate, sensitive, and patient.

I think things always happen for a reason, or at least that you can use all things for good with the right motivation. I told Alan this diagnosis could be a whole new purpose for him. By helping himself he could help countless others who don't know where to start, or don't know what to do, and that he could not only be compassionate but possibly pave the way for others.

He has done that for many people. Not just people with MS but those with cancer, colitis, and so much more. He was willing to research anything for anyone because he knew how helpful it could be and how lost people can feel. We don't all have the same gifts and talents, but when we use the ones we have to help others — well, that's truly what it's all about, and I couldn't be prouder of him.

THERE'S PLENTY OF HELP LOCALLY — JUST ASK

We really are so very fortunate in our society. There are all kinds of societies, associations, foundations, support groups, and counseling programs available to us. The kinds of help and support required vary with each different diagnosis, and the specifics of what's available to you depend on where you live. But it's out there.

The best way to find out about what's available to you once you're diagnosed is to start with your doctors. Start with a specialist in what you "have." Typically they have an up-to-date list of options for help and support and may well participate in some of them with their patients.

Most family doctors or GPs are also aware of the various programs. In many cases, because you have a long-standing relationship with your family doctor, they may be able to direct you to programs or people they have heard good things about.

Some doctors are also willing to refer you to other patients who live in your area and are willing to chat with you one on one. This can be a fantastic resource. But please remember: Don't take the opinions of any one doctor or patient as the complete story. The more input you get, the better able you will be to make good decisions for yourself.

FIVE

NAVIGATING THE
HEALTHCARE PROCESS

Doctors give drugs of which they know little,
into bodies, of which they know less,
for diseases of which they know nothing at all.
— VOLTAIRE

MANY OF US become anxious about losing our jobs or becoming
uninsurable once we are labeled with a debilitating or degenerative
disease or condition. There are lots of articles and books (along with
television specials) dealing with the absolute crime this represents.
It clearly demonstrates a weakness in the medical system and the
way we as a society view and deal with serious illness.

I'm going to avoid getting into details about the complicated
situation of HMO- or government-supplied medicine. It's too specific
to where you live, who you are, and what you've got (illness-wise and
money-wise).

One important point is that many of the statistics on how many
people have a specific disease or illness are just plain wrong. They
are often understated and therefore misleading. That's because many

patients stop the diagnostic process once it becomes evident a diagnosis is coming that may result in social or financial (including insurance) trouble. They simply don't want to be "labeled" forevermore. The numbers are also wrong because there is no uniform procedure for reporting many illnesses, and because many diagnoses are very subjective, which leaves lots of room for uncertainty. This means some of the decisions made by governments, insurance companies, and doctors (especially those involved in research) are based on bad information. These numbers also have an impact on drug pricing and research and are at the root of some of the biggest problems plaguing the medical and insurance systems.

If the number of people affected by a condition or illness is understated, how can the healthcare system ever be adequately prepared to meet the needs of such people, or give proper priority to looking for treatments or cures? Let's face it, if everyone thinks illness or disease affects a relatively small number of people — say, 1% of the population versus 10% — where are research and support dollars going to go?

Lack of current and accurate statistics about who has what leads to confusion and frustration, particularly for newly diagnosed or almost diagnosed patients and their families.

This is where some clinics, societies, hospital-related programs, your insurance company, and the like can be helpful, at least in narrowing down what may or may not be available to you.

What's really important to you at this stage — and this is the focus of this chapter — are the doctors and drugs that pertain to you directly. This chapter shows you how they can and should be managed directly by you. It shows you how to navigate the healthcare system.

THE BAD NEWS ABOUT SPECIALIZATION

The more medical science learns and the more refined the investigative tools of science become, the greater the amount of information a doctor needs to know. For this reason many doctors are becoming more and more specialized. After all, this makes the amount of information they need to absorb more manageable for them.

But apparently that's not the only reason to specialize. Another is that the greater the number of doctors involved in a case, the less likely any one of them will be sued individually. When many doctors are involved, which one do you blame if things go wrong? By specializing in smaller and smaller areas, doctors are forced to involve other doctors in your case for their diagnostic contribution. Not only does this tend to minimize their legal exposure, it also contributes to the ever-increasing costs of medical care and wait times for patients.

That statement will make some doctors mad, and it should.

Getting the best diagnosis possible seems to have become a lot more about money (including payments to and disputes with insurance companies or applicable institutions), the law, and politics (both governmental and professional) than about the patient.

All these parties, plus medicine in general, need to come to some kind of understanding for the sake of all patients. I believe medical lawsuits typically hurt way more patients than they help. Often the only real winners in these suits are the attorneys involved and the surviving family members. It is often too late for the patient. I am talking more about malpractice here than about all the prescription-related suits that are so often in the news, which are another matter entirely. Perhaps there should be a cap on what attorneys can make on a medically related suit or maybe a "flat rate."

When big dollars are involved, there's too much incentive for big abuse.

Certainly when a mistake is made or negligence occurs, the patient should be cared for legally, but doctors need to be encouraged to provide patients with *all* the options and to get more involved with a patient's diagnosis and choice of ongoing care. The only way that's going to happen is if we find ways to decrease their liability. That would help them talk and think about things above and beyond the standard of care. After all, viable options, based on their use by proactive patients and out-of-the-box docs (I'll get to them later, in chapter eight), sometimes *become* the next standard of care. For this to happen, fear of liability has to be decreased. Protection for doctors from frivolous suits and the unrealistic costs of malpractice insurance needs to be a high priority. I have often wondered lately what our world would be like if doctors only got paid when we were healthy.

THE GOOD NEWS ABOUT SPECIALIZATION

But there's good news about specialization, too.

If you have a condition that can be readily diagnosed, and see the right specialist at the right time, you can get a reasonably accurate diagnosis early on. You may be one of the lucky ones who, first time out, get a definitive diagnosis that proves to be correct long-term.

This may minimize any damage caused by your condition and get you started on a good course of treatment quickly.

Also, specialization can be beneficial when it comes to surgery. I'd rather be operated on by a surgeon who does a select few surgeries day in and day out than by one who has to refresh their memory about the procedure before cutting me open.

WORKING THE SYSTEM

Healthcare systems try to make it difficult for us to direct the quantity and quality of care and attention we receive. No doubt this comes back to cost, or more specifically cost savings, because often the number one question is, "Who pays?" Number two is, "How much?" Most people who are lucky enough to have access to supplemented health care know that their individual opinions or desires generally have little bearing on the choices available to them through HMOs, insurance companies, and (in countries like Canada) government-sponsored facilities. Choices need to come from or be refereed by doctors and often need to be "approved." After all, what do most patients know about medicine or health? Patients always want the best of whatever is available. If you were or are the patient, wouldn't you? But who's going to pay?

This is why if things really go wrong and you know you're headed for a scary diagnosis, you need to take control of your situation fast. Typically, being pleasant but firm is best, but if you do feel you need to "lose it" in order to get someone's attention, try to make it about you, your care, and your condition. Don't dump on the doctors (or anyone else) or get personal. Doctors and hospitals tend to be small, tight-knit communities, so it's best for you to practice the "do unto others" thing as much as possible. Try to be nice, even though you may be ready to scream.

Your doctors need to see you as an individual, not as just another one of their patients. It is far too easy for doctors, especially specialists, to lump all similarly diagnosed patients into groups. Since many diagnoses are truly best guesses, you want to make sure you are "visible" enough to keep your doctor focused on you, your symptoms, and your case, not on the group you've been slotted into.

It's important to connect, personally, with all of your doctors. You don't have to make them like you, although that wouldn't hurt, but you do need to get them and keep them interested in you and your problem. The more interested they are, the more information they are likely to gather on you and the more time they are likely to spend contemplating your case and discussing it with you.

If you feel, after the first couple of visits, that a doctor isn't interested in you, then you need to try harder, change tactics, or get another doctor. A credible patient, one who asks good questions and seems to be on the ball, often has an advantage over the submissive patient. This is true not only in terms of getting attention but also in terms of increasing your chances of a better outcome.

Perhaps the worst thing for you, the patient, is confusion. With some symptoms you could receive a different diagnosis from just about every specialist you see. After all, when doctors are focused on a limited view of you and your symptoms, they're more likely to see a condition within their area of expertise, especially when observation and interpretation are the main diagnostic tools being used.

Many patients get passed around from one specialist to another when their problem isn't obvious. One reason for this is that doctors tend not to look at the patient as a whole. They don't even try to connect the dots, because any dot outside their specialization is a dot outside the picture they're looking at or comfortable with. They focus on the part of the person they specialize in.

Referrals to specialists may be necessary, but typically tend to frustrate and stress out the patient. Try to keep calm, and be patient. This will be easier to do if you know you're being proactive and have some sense of what's happening and why.

As for the communication of information about you and your case between specialists (and all doctors), it generally stinks.

This is especially true if you're not being sent for a second opinion, but to another, different kind of specialist. Information seems to flow better with second opinions, perhaps because one doctor is sort of checking the work of another in the same field.

This is why you should ask for copies of all tests, reports, and pictures that become part of your case. You may be told you can't have some of these, but that doesn't seem to happen that much any more. Medical tests, reports, and records about you should be available to you. You may occasionally have to pay some fees for copies, but it's worth it.

I got copies of everything, and I do mean everything, and put them in three-ring binders. I kept a calendar of when I had what done to me and who ordered it. I carried all that stuff around with me most of the time. It was amazing how often the doctors I was referred to had incomplete and occasionally incorrect information. Don't assume anything. When it comes to your medical information, you want each and every doctor to have it all and in its most current form.

As I have observed the healthcare system through the lens of my own case, I have often wondered why specialists in a clinical setting don't work more often as teams. That way they could confer and work together to make the best possible choices for the patient, cutting time and expense in the process.

Things are changing slowly. There are a growing number of clinics and professional practices with specialists working together. However, they are the exception rather than the rule.

"BEST SPECIALISTS"

In my Internet research, following my diagnosis, I came across an article using the phrase "scary diagnosis" and of course read it. This led me to a website that specializes in offering second opinions and other services from doctors they consider the best. The site, www.BestDoctors.com, has both a u.s. and a Canadian section. Although I have no first-hand experience with these folks, I'm presenting this as an example of what is currently available to you if you look. This site does give clues to where the future of care is going. An Internet search will provide additional competitive choices.

Following is some material from the Canadian part of the site. I have footnoted the exact web pages that were in use when I wrote this.

INTERCONSULTATION™

An in-depth review of your medical files to assist in the development and confirmation of the diagnosis and to help develop a treatment plan. You and your physicians will have access to the latest technologies and opinions of world-class specialists. With a fast and detailed turnaround of results, the InterConsultation process can reduce potentially serious complications that can result from a misdiagnosis and help your treating physician determine the proper course of action.[5]

FINDBESTDOC™

Sometimes the medical care required for a specific diagnosis goes beyond borders. That's when our exclusive global database of more than 50,000 specialists proves to be an invaluable resource for you, your physician and your family.

Your Personal Advocate will ask what is most important to you. Is it geographic location, the cost or availability of a specialist?

Best Doctors will conduct a search based on your answers.

We'll provide you with a detailed report containing

---

5   http://www.bestdoctors.com/canada/interconsultation.php

information on up to three specialists including their educational background and training, as well as their relevant experience to your particular case. The report even indicates when these specialists would be available to see you.

If you decide to see one of the best doctors in Canada, we'll provide our report to you and your local family physician so they can make a referral. Should you choose to go outside of Canada for treatment, our concierge service will book all of your appointments and even take care of your travel arrangements.

Helping you find the best doctors and treatment in the world.

That's our commitment.[6]

FINDBESTCARE™

If you decide that you are going to be treated by a physician identified by Best Doctors, FindBestCare helps take the worry out of making travel arrangements for you and your family, reducing stress so you can concentrate on getting well again.

The FindBestCare program includes a full concierge service to help make all arrangements such as booking airfare, hotel accommodations, ground transportation, translation services, medical appointments, hospital admissions, etc.[*]

If you choose to go to the United States for medical care, Best Doctors also manages a cost containment process to help ensure you are not overcharged or billed incorrectly. We'll provide you with a full report outlining all the charges, what discounts were applied, and the final amount to be paid.

FindBestCare also provides case management services to respond to any inquiries that you or family members may have

---

6   http://www.bestdoctors.com/canada/findbestdoc.php

during the treatment process.

Members are responsible for all costs related to treatment, travel and lodging.[7]

DRUGS ALONE ARE THE EASY WAY OUT

When it comes to treating patients, and especially kids, drugs all too often seem the easy answer. Drugs typically focus on symptoms, because most of the time we know so little about the actual causes, we haven't developed drugs to counteract them. In what follows, I'll use the term "drugs" to mean both prescription and over-the-counter.

Aren't there options other than, or in addition to, drugs?

And if so, why do they seem to be last on the list?

Modern medicine focuses on drugs and operations or procedures, and this focus has also become a media favorite, as evidenced by the endless medical shows and special reports. It's understandable, then, that these are most sought after by patients. In fact, that's what patients have come to expect or even demand. But why?

Why does it often seem that some of the other choices for preventing or addressing illness and disease are targets for vilification, even though they may be no better or worse than mainstream choices?

Drugs and surgery are certainly the tools doctors are most trained to use. Often they are also the most expensive routes to take, even though results are less impressive than one might expect. (It should be noted that research is often focused more on treatment than on cause and cure.)

---

7   http://www.bestdoctors.com/canada/findbestcare.php

One can't help wonder, given the amount of money spent researching conditions like cancer, heart disease, and MS, why so little progress is being made. It seems that the more we try to figure out how to be healthy, the more health problems materialize. So what do we do, where do we start, and to whom do we turn? Let's look at some statistics and see if they match how you view modern medicine.

The following is a summary, by Joseph Mercola, M.D., of an article in the *Journal of American Medical Association*. I came across this on Dr. Mercola's website, www.mercola.com.

Doctors Are the Third Leading Cause of Death in the US, Causing 250,000 Deaths Every Year

This article in the *Journal of the American Medical Association* (JAMA) is the best article I have ever seen written in the published literature documenting the tragedy of the traditional medical paradigm.

This information is a followup of the Institute of Medicine report which hit the papers in December of last year, but the data [were] hard to reference as [they were] not in peer-reviewed journals. Now it is published in JAMA which is the most widely circulated medical periodical in the world.

The author is Dr. Barbara Starfield of the Johns Hopkins School of Hygiene and Public Health and she describes how the US health care system may contribute to poor health.

ALL THESE ARE DEATHS PER YEAR:

- 12,000 — unnecessary surgery
- 7,000 — medication errors in hospitals
- 20,000 — other errors in hospitals
- 80,000 — infections in hospitals

- 106,000 — non-error, negative effects of drugs

These total to 250,000 deaths per year from iatrogenic causes.

What does the word iatrogenic mean? This term is defined as induced in a patient by a physician's activity, manner, or therapy. Used especially of a complication of treatment.

Dr. Starfield offers several warnings in interpreting these numbers:

First, most of the data are derived from studies in hospitalized patients.

Second, these estimates are for deaths only and do not include negative effects that are associated with disability or discomfort.

Third, the estimates of death due to error are lower than those in the IOM report.

If the higher estimates are used, the deaths due to iatrogenic causes would range from 230,000 to 284,000. In any case, 225,000 deaths per year constitutes the third leading cause of death in the United States, after deaths from heart disease and cancer. Even if these figures are overestimated, there is a wide margin between these numbers of deaths and the next leading cause of death (cerebrovascular disease).

Another analysis concluded that between 4% and 18% of consecutive patients experience negative effects in outpatient settings, with:

- 116 million extra physician visits
- 77 million extra prescriptions
- 17 million emergency department visits
- 8 million hospitalizations
- 3 million long-term admissions
- 199,000 additional deaths
- $77 billion in extra costs

The high cost of the health care system is considered to be a deficit, but seems to be tolerated under the assumption that better health results from more expensive care.

However, evidence from a few studies indicates that as many as 20% to 30% of patients receive inappropriate care.

An estimated 44,000 to 98,000 among them die each year as a result of medical errors.

This might be tolerated if it resulted in better health, but does it? Of 13 countries in a recent comparison, the United States ranks an average of 12th (second from the bottom) for 16 available health indicators. More specifically, the ranking of the US on several indicators was:

- 13th (last) for low-birth-weight percentages
- 13th for neonatal mortality and infant mortality overall
- 11th for postneonatal mortality
- 13th for years of potential life lost (excluding external causes)
- 11th for life expectancy at 1 year for females, 12th for males
- 10th for life expectancy at 15 years for females, 12th for males
- 10th for life expectancy at 40 years for females, 9th for males
- 7th for life expectancy at 65 years for females, 7th for males
- 3rd for life expectancy at 80 years for females, 3rd for males
- 10th for age-adjusted mortality

The poor performance of the US was recently confirmed by a World Health Organization study, which used different data and ranked the United States as 15th among 25 industrialized countries.

There is a perception that the American public "behaves badly" by smoking, drinking, and perpetrating violence. However the data [do] not support this assertion.

The proportion of females who smoke ranges from 14% in

Japan to 41% in Denmark; in the United States, it is 24% (fifth best). For males, the range is from 26% in Sweden to 61% in Japan; it is 28% in the United States (third best).

The US ranks fifth best for alcoholic beverage consumption.

The US has relatively low consumption of animal fats (fifth lowest in men aged 55–64 years in 20 industrialized countries) and the third lowest mean cholesterol concentrations among men aged 50 to 70 years among 13 industrialized countries.

These estimates of death due to error are lower than those in a recent Institute of Medicine report, and if the higher estimates are used, the deaths due to iatrogenic causes would range from 230,000 to 284,000.

Even at the lower estimate of 225,000 deaths per year, this constitutes the third leading cause of death in the US, following heart disease and cancer.

Lack of technology is certainly not a contributing factor to the US's low ranking.

Among 29 countries, the United States is second only to Japan in the availability of magnetic resonance imaging units and computed tomography scanners per million population.

Japan, however, ranks highest on health, whereas the US ranks among the lowest.

It is possible that the high use of technology in Japan is limited to diagnostic technology not matched by high rates of treatment, whereas in the US, high use of diagnostic technology may be linked to more treatment.

Supporting this possibility are data showing that the number of employees per bed (full-time equivalents) in the United States is highest among the countries ranked, whereas they are very low in Japan, far lower than can be accounted for by the common practice of having family members rather than hospital staff provide the amenities of hospital care.[8]

Do these statistics fit comfortably into your current picture of drugs and their use?

THE TREATMENT, NOT THE CURE

It stands to reason that if we don't know what caused an illness or condition to begin with, figuring out how to treat it is going to be quite the challenge.

It appears this is one reason why treatments focus on specific symptoms rather than on fixing or curing the problem.

At least for the cynical or suspicious, or perhaps the business-savvy among us, there's another reason the focus rarely seems to be on a cure: It's far more profitable to address symptoms than to search for cures.

That's the reality behind the common statement that "the money is in the treatment not the cure." To some extent this is true, but in all fairness there's a lot more to it. It's important to acknowledge that patients themselves are often more focused on their symptoms and dealing with them than on a cure. That's how we seem to have been trained to think.

We become preoccupied with what we're dealing with day by day. We're all held back from the important issues of health and wellness by our short-sighted desire for quick fixes and physical comfort. It probably takes most of us a relatively long time to build up all the necessary ingredients to get really sick, yet we're programmed to want to be fixed overnight. In all likelihood, at least short-term,

---

8   http://www.mercola.com/2000/jul/30/doctors_death.htm

it's going to take a major change in our perspective for us to be ready to work with longer-term fixes or cures.

Let's take a quick look, from a business perspective, at the way the "system" dictates how things work in the world of medicine.

The healthcare and pharmaceutical industries are mammoth in North America (and worldwide). They employ massive numbers of people, pay big taxes, and spend big money on ads and lobbying governments.

Suppose large numbers of folks were to get well. What would the financial, social, and political impact of this be on our economies, the stock market, and politics with all its related lobbying? Think of all the people who would lose their jobs if hospitals and doctors weren't busy, people stopped taking so many drugs, and insurance and government agencies didn't have to process the mountains of paper they do currently, all because people weren't sick.

I'm not saying that all the good folks who work in medicine, the pharmaceutical industry, or our governments don't want us healthy. I'm saying that the sheer size of healthcare and related insurance and drug companies, and the amount of money involved, tend to slow down or otherwise affect how things work.

It's something at least to think about. It certainly affects those of us dealing with a scary diagnosis, from the very start of our problem and on an ongoing basis.

Here's something else to think about: the stem cell controversy. What if stem cell research ends up making treatments or cures available for a wide range of illnesses and conditions? What if millions of people could get well almost overnight? Is fear of the impact this would have on economies worldwide behind the antagonism toward stem cell research in North America? (I'm not speaking here about the ethical issues, which apply only to one type of stem cell — embryonic.)

Nothing like a good conspiracy theory. In any case, any mainstream beneficial effects of stem cell research are still a ways off. Drugs remain the primary tool.

Doctors are armed with basically two tools: medications and operations. I think it's fair to say that most of us expect at least one prescription when we visit a doctor. If we don't get a prescription, then why did we go? What else does a doctor typically do to treat us other than give us a quick examination and ask *us* what's wrong?

We expect a prescription or two at the very least, don't we? We're probably hoping not to hear the word "operation."

A great example of the marketing material used by doctors and drug companies telling only part of the story was when I researched the CRAB drugs for treating MS.

The marketing material indicated that I could expect about a 30% reduction in "attacks" through regular injections of any of these drugs. That meant if I was having three MS attacks a year, I could expect, on average, a decrease of one attack a year. Two attacks is a better number than three, but still not good as far as I'm concerned.

Further reading on medical sites and from reports of clinical trials revealed to me that the placebo used during most of the clinical trials often resulted in a 20–25% reduction in attacks. That meant that the drugs performed only 5–10% better than the placebo (probably saline or something similar). It seemed to me I could almost get the same reduction in attacks from the placebo as from the expensive drug with a scary list of side effects.

What do you think about that? I wasn't impressed. This brings up the apparent effectiveness of placebos, which is an interesting subject in itself. Placebos seem to work because we think they'll work. There's no doubt we affect how we feel by what we think. The whole mind/body connection has been demonstrated repeatedly but overall remains neglected. (We'll talk a bit more about this later.)

Not sure about what I'm saying about why I chose not to use a CRAB drug? Not sure my information is correct? Prove it to yourself by doing an Internet search for "Avonex placebo" or placebos associated with any of the other CRAB drugs (Copaxone, Rebif, Betaserone). It will make for interesting reading, I assure you. The numbers may vary a bit from site to site or from study to study, but performance compared with a placebo remains about the same.

I'm not saying one or all of the CRAB drugs should not be considered as an option for you if you have been given an MS diagnosis. I am saying that I concluded, based on my own basic risk-versus-reward analysis and the issues we've discussed, that it was not an attractive option for me. At least not now.

PATIENT FEEDBACK

The research I conducted was only part of why I decided not to inject a CRAB drug.

Feedback and comments written by other patients who had used some or even all of the CRAB drugs were a factor, too. I found most of this material in user groups on the Internet, and often followed it up with direct contact via email.

This type of feedback from other patients, typically referred to as anecdotal evidence, should be factored into everyone's decision-making process. Some folks, particularly doctors and drug companies, often consider anecdotal evidence pretty much useless — unless, of course, it happens to support their position or claim. Personally,

I have come to understand that learning from the experience of others dealing with similar issues can provide some valuable clues and insights. It can give us the information we need in order to come up with good questions. It is then up to each one of us to get the answers that will help us make the best decisions for us.

A NEW DAY FOR ALL KINDS OF MEDICINE

As I've said before, I have nothing against doctors. I admire and appreciate them. That said, there's always room for improvement. As a patient who is proactive and learning daily about what's happening to me and about some of the issues and options that may have an impact on me, I can see the need for reflection and change. Not just on the part of the professionals and services dedicated to helping patients, but on the part of patients, too.

Several medical limitations have become obvious to me through my medical ordeal and adventure.

As mentioned, most medical doctors are trained in and focus on two specific treatment modalities: drugs and operations.

Many times, if not most times, one or both of these treatment modalities will be at least somewhat helpful to the patient. It's what doctors know and what patients have come to expect.

But these two treatment modalities are not the only ones available. They are the most common and mainstream, but that doesn't mean other choices cannot or will not have some positive impact.

I'm talking about alternative treatments or alternative medicine. (This subject will be discussed in greater detail in chapter eight.) Many doctors are quick to point out that these are often unregulated, have little in the way of proof (few clinical trials), are too simple, or are too far outside their comfort zones — based on their education, training, and experience — for them to be able to support or condone their use.

And quite frankly, they are generally too busy or too focused on what they know (or believe they know) to be willing to even consider alternative treatments, regardless of the evidence (anecdotal or clinical). I use the term "alternative treatments" not only for approaches regular doctors typically refuse to use, but also for ones they or other doctors may use but are uncomfortable with. Alternative treatments and alternative medicine are huge subjects. To simplify things, I am using "alternative treatments" to refer to things that may be used by some medical doctors but are not typically part of their regular training or in general use by their peers.

Doctors are heavily influenced by the various professional groups they belong to (like the American Medical Association) and the pharmaceutical and medical companies making the drugs, equipment, and tools they are trained to work with. Both these groups are either directly or indirectly responsible for education (both initial and ongoing) and for providing the direction that ends up being the position and focus of many doctors.

Doctors are exposed to drug company representatives and their marketing material (and samples) at their offices and at conferences and seminars. Is it any wonder the sponsors of their continuing education are the primary influence on their belief system?

Clinical evidence is based on testing — the so-called clinical trial. It's often presented as absolute fact, but how factual are clinical trials?

Anecdotal evidence, meanwhile, is basically a bunch of patients saying ("claiming") that something is helpful or "works" for them.

As a patient, and one not satisfied with the drug options available to me for MS, I am finding there often are several ways to address a health issue. I'm hoping, based on all we have talked about so far, that you're convinced or inspired to explore your options for yourself. Always do some checking yourself regardless of who is telling you what.

Here's an example of choosing treatments other than drugs.

When I was in my late 30s, a doctor whom I considered very good at what he did questioned why I was seeing a chiropractor for degenerative discs in my neck. He knew I had suffered from pain related to these discs for years. Even I could look at the x-rays and see the problem clearly.

This doctor asked me why I would risk seeing a chiropractor when he could continue to prescribe drugs for me — an anti-inflammatory and a muscle relaxant — that would control my problem over time. I explained that the muscle relaxant made me dopey and that I was concerned about the long-term effects of the anti-inflammatory drugs.

I also explained that when my neck was "out," I typically experienced relief within a day or two of visiting the chiropractor versus within a week or two of starting on the drugs — unless I took lots of pain killers, which made me useless for dealing with life in general.

He just didn't believe in chiropractic manipulation, or was afraid of it, or simply wouldn't accept it.

Now, this was more than 15 years ago, but it's indicative of how doctors look at "alternatives" even today. Some may argue chiropractors are not alternative therapists, but not this M.D.

And here's a quick example of how what was unacceptable yesterday is good medicine today.

It wasn't long ago that many North American doctors didn't

believe in the efficacy of acupuncture. Today it is frequently used and taught in hospitals, particularly as a replacement for or supplement to local anesthesia in some operations and in pain management.

Do we now, all of a sudden, understand how acupuncture works, where we didn't before? No, not really.

What is alternative today may well be mainstream tomorrow. When you're the one who's ill, you need to be open-minded, even if your doctors aren't.

I am not suggesting you ignore your doctors. Quite the contrary.

I am alerting you to the fact that it's up to you and not them to search, research, and ask the right questions. Taking responsibility is key to taking charge, to being productively proactive.

CLINICAL TRIALS

Clinical trials are used and sometimes abused by those selling a concept or product. Here's why.

These trials are often paid for by the drug company that holds the patents on the drugs being "tested." The results of the trials may then help them sell those drugs. These trials can be expensive.

In general, the reporting of results of clinical trials is controlled by the companies that do the trials (and own the drugs), and the reports are their property. This means the public typically sees the results of successful trials only. In theory, a drug could perform poorly in 19 trials and well in the 20th and we would hear only about the good one. The trials are typically redesigned between tries, so given enough time and testing it may be possible for almost any drug to "pass" a trial.

Is the clinical trial concept that much better than anecdotal evidence? One would think so, except that some very serious questions have been raised about these trials by some very important folks.

Whether the clinical trial process is broken or not is a big issue and an interesting one. Do some research and reading about clinical trials and examine whether they really mean what you think they mean. I'm certain you'll be very surprised. Do a quick search with your search engine using "clinical trials" and "fraud" or "issues" (or similar key words) and do some reading. Dr. Mercola's website has an interesting analysis of the book *The Truth About Drug Companies: How They Deceive Us and What to Do About It.*[9] The book is written by Dr. Marcia Angell, a member of Harvard Medical School's Department of Social Medicine and a former editor of the *New England Journal of Medicine.*

Clinical trials have a special place in my heart (well, in my mind anyway) because I came across a drug I was interested in taking while I was in an MS user group. It seemed to be getting some very positive commentary. In other words, good anecdotal evidence was being presented. (LDN and my experience with it are discussed in detail in chapter nine.)

Although this drug, referred to as LDN, was FDA-approved, it was not approved or tested for MS. That would require clinical trials. Why wouldn't the manufacturers of LDN pay for these trials if people with MS were starting to take it and reporting favorable results? A Harvard graduate and well-published neurologist practicing in Manhattan has been prescribing it with growing success for around 20 years.

So why no trials?

---

9   http://mercola.com/2004/aug/25/drug_companies.htm

Well, simply put, LDN is apparently too old and too cheap. It costs me less than a dollar a day — peanuts compared with prices charged for "approved" MS drugs. It has no patent protection. In other words, since the drug companies see no prospect of big profits from the drug, it is simply not cost-effective to put money into testing its effects on MS and getting it approved for MS. The pharmaceutical companies can't make serious money on a cheap drug that is past patent protection and available as a generic, compared with what they can make on more expensive and "younger" (still patent-protected) drugs.

Fire up your search engines and do some reading. The good news is that things may be changing with respect to this drug. There are some clinical trials of LDN happening and others being considered — one on LDN and Crohn's disease, a couple on MS, and some others. Some of them are happening because universities got involved, others because LDN users are banding together and raising money.

DRUG TESTING

The FDA in the U.S. (which, depending on where you live and what drugs you are taking, you may or may not feel is the pertinent group) requires certain things to be done before a drug can be approved for general use.

With the very public failure of several drugs recently (and with a long list of other perhaps less public failures over many years), the entire process of testing and approval is being questioned.

The truth is that there is simply no perfect way to test new drugs. Yet another statement most readers won't like, but it's true.

There are just too many variables. In order to conduct perfect tests, you'd need patients with the same genetics, diets, environments, other medications, lifestyles, and even personalities (so they have similar levels of stress). Come to think of it, clones would be perfect for these tests — no, we're not going there.

Not only are the tests dicey because of all the human variables involved, but they often aren't even performed on humans — they start with animals. Unless the human version of the disease in question can be transferred to animals, the animals are given diseases that approximate or mimic the human versions. How close are the animal versions? Given such approximations, how much will a rabbit or mouse's response to a drug tell us about the response of humans who have the actual disease?

So why are drugs and drug testing all of a sudden such big issues in the news and otherwise?

Because of the speed and reach of today's communications technologies and the public's increased desire for information. This makes it very difficult to keep everyone in the dark about something like drug trials, although some would argue there is just too much information to make any sense of it.

Another part of the controversy is the amount of money involved.

It is estimated that total sales of the cholesterol medication Lipitor, *in one year*, are between $10 billion and $12 billion U.S.

So is the drug industry today's Evil Empire? Some would say yes. I cut the drug companies a little slack because I think most of the time they're playing the game the best they can.

Are rules being stretched and bent? Yes.

But since the drug companies serve two masters, the shareholders and the drug users, can we really blame them for testing and marketing drugs that have the best chance of economic success? If the rules were different, the game would be different and we might all feel different about the pharmaceutical industry.

DRUG COMMERCIALS

What about all those drug commercials on television? You know the ones I mean. The ones that use the formula, "Ask your doctor about xxxxx." This is clever. If patients come at their doctors inquiring about specific drugs, the doctors are going to feel obligated to prescribe those drugs.

Often a significant part of the commercials is a recitation of a long list of side effects, which is required by law.

Half the time the ads don't even say what the drugs are for.

What's all that about? Does it make sense coming from an industry that's supposed to be all about ethics?

And what went into deciding that prescription drugs need to be marketed directly to the public through a prime-time sales pitch? Making information available to patients — for instance, on websites — is one thing. Bombarding people with partial information is another. When these ads encourage patients to ask their doctors about the drugs, are they playing on the public's suspicion that doctors are not paying attention to their specific needs as patients?

By all means, ask your doctor questions — not after hearing the name of a drug in a vague commercial but after you've done your homework. Only by doing the latter will you be able to ask intelligent questions that pertain to your issues.

What's really odd is that often only a small part of a drug company's budget is spent on research, with much more spent on advertising. It's not as if you can just go out and buy the drugs. You need to see a doctor to get them. That's why the companies need you to ask your doctor about their drugs.

Your doctor should be figuring out what's best to prescribe to you before you need to ask. If not, maybe you should be looking for another doctor, don't you think?

I am not contradicting myself here. You still need to be proactive and ask questions. You still need to be doing the research. I am simply warning you not to waste precious time and effort on things that may have little or nothing to do with your problem or its solution.

I just can't make any real sense out of "dealing prescription drugs" on television. Good grief, kids are watching these ads. What do you think is going through their impressionable minds as they see them? One of the biggest problems associated with kids and drug abuse is the recreational use of prescription drugs, not illegal ones. Think about that, and all it implies.

A CASE IN POINT: POT

Marijuana, which earlier I admitted to smoking in my misspent youth, kept popping up as I did my homework looking for things that might help me feel better and get better. I know some of you are smiling, but pot does have some medicinal uses that simply can't be denied.

There's a growing acceptance of pot as a legitimate prescription drug and there are places or situations where doctors can in fact prescribe it.

Some clinical trials and certainly lots of anecdotal evidence indicate that, in some cases, pot performs better than other choices for certain conditions, such as ones involving nausea, some kinds of pain, glaucoma, and MS.

If you search the Internet for information on "marijuana" in combination with "chemotherapy," "radiation," "AIDS," "MS," or "medicinal uses," you'll be reading for days.

Certainly the anecdotal evidence confirms marijuana's efficacy. The problem with its widespread medicinal use stems from how easy it is to grow the stuff and its popularity as an illegal "recreational" drug.

Pot grows like a weed because it is a weed — one that anyone can grow, both indoors and out. This makes it tough for anyone to make money on legalized pot.

That's simply a fact, and it's why it continues to be irrationally controlled for medicinal use. This probably wouldn't be the case if someone could figure out how to make it a revenue generator for big business, like alcohol or cigarettes. My guess is it would be for sale tomorrow if it weren't so damn easy to grow and smoke. And I bet tobacco would be treated like pot if it was as easy to grow.

I want to make it clear that I am not encouraging anyone to use pot recreationally, nor am I encouraging anyone to break the law.

I do find it ironic that because I have been diagnosed with MS I can actually get the stuff legally, by prescription. Finding a doctor willing to prescribe it is another story, however. My first neurologist said he would never write a prescription for it because he didn't want to become known as a "marijuana doctor." That's another reason why he's no longer my doctor. When doctors are more concerned about what others think of them than about what might be best for you, it's time for you to move on.

I don't have a prescription for pot, nor do I use it illegally. Thankfully, my symptoms are such that I don't need it. I have corresponded with a couple of people who have used medical marijuana. A common comment is that it is so processed and inconvenient to get that many if not most end up going back to buying it or growing it illegally. Perhaps it's time the medical profession and society took a good hard look at the political and social issues involved and did the right thing for patients who need the drugs.

Montel Williams, the famous talk show host, has MS and admits to using pot on a fairly regular basis. He speaks out about it often, has written several books on it, and works to see it legalized for medicinal use. Have a look at his website and books.

The fact that clinical trials say it's okay, some governments say it's okay, and patients say it works better than anything else for some symptoms (better even than some pretty serious prescription meds that I could get if I needed them) evidently means nothing to some doctors and politicians and segments of the public. I'm guessing that would change overnight if *they* got sick and thought it could help *them*.

I just can't get over how willing most doctors are to prescribe much "harder" and far more dangerous drugs with respect to side effects and addiction issues than marijuana simply because they're manufactured, pharmaceutical drugs. I think it's a very sad commentary on our priorities as a society — that we're more interested in money and politics than in what's best for patients. Put that in your pipe and smoke it.

BEING PROACTIVE

We've talked a lot about doctors because they are a huge part of the process associated with identifying and dealing with a scary diagnosis. What you actually end up doing after going through the process is where being productively proactive comes in.

Here, for example, is a quick summary of what I did. (Some of what follows has been discussed above; the rest will be dealt with in more detail later in the book.)

- I researched my symptoms and diagnosis and had a hard look at any and all other things my symptoms might indicate, with the goal of eliminating other potential diagnoses.
- I got copies of anything and everything related to my research, and the testing done on me, and built a file that I carried with me. That file included a calendar so I could remember and track what was happening and when. I used it to "educate" and update, when necessary, any doctors I was scheduled to see.
- I accepted that I had an ongoing health issue and decided I was going to be proactive and take control.
- I had my mercury fillings removed. I began several procedures to remove the mercury from my body, focusing especially on chelation. I started studying diet, nutrition, and dental health as they relate to wellness. I started eating differently.
- I tried different supplements and began an exercise program. I found a doctor willing to work with me. He was willing to order many of the tests I wanted done based on my research, and added some of his own. The goal was to look for additional "clues" and eliminate other potential diagnoses.
- I allowed myself to sleep at least eight to ten hours a day. I made every effort to remove as many of the most stressful things from my daily life as possible.
- I made some kind of exercise a daily priority, even if it was only minimal at the start.
- I played more guitar — something I had been teaching myself to do for a few years. I played more golf. Yes, I know both guitar and golf can be stressful, but I try to control myself.
- I stopped saying, "I have MS." I realized I didn't have MS — I had a diagnosis of MS. I am not MS and if it really exists as a true

disease it is not going to define who I am. I am a living, breathing, ever-changing individual. I became focused on changing for the better.

SIX

NAVIGATING THE
INTERNET FOR ANSWERS

When I took office, only high energy physicists
had ever heard of what is called the World Wide Web ...
Now even my cat has its own page.
— BILL CLINTON

USING A COMPUTER and searching the Internet is a key part of my story and needs to be a key part of yours.

Since the goal here is not to teach you how to use a computer but to help you sift through the vast mountain of information to get to the stuff that will help you, I offer you, in this chapter, some basic knowledge.

You may be new to computers or have only limited exposure to them. There's nothing to be afraid of. It may be best to find pretty much any kid to teach you the basics.

In addition to computers being a great tool for doing research, they open up whole new worlds of communication through email and instant messaging. This can certainly be a tremendous aid to you if you're dealing with a scary diagnosis. For one thing, it will allow you to easily communicate with others who have similar issues.

The ability to ask and answers questions is a tremendous asset. You're never alone when you have access to the Internet. Some may think that's not a good thing (especially for unsupervised children), but when you're ill, it's irreplaceable.

It should also be noted that a computer can open up new worlds of entertainment to you and give you an easy way to begin keeping records. It also allows you to easily begin writing about what you're going through — something that is a help to many.

HOW TO SEARCH THE INTERNET

Following is a very brief description of how to search the Internet.

To do so, you need a computer with Internet access. Some wireless devices, including some cellular telephones, have Internet capability. But for the kind of searching you'll need and want to be doing, a computer attached to a printer works best.

It would be best to have a high-speed connection of some kind. Currently cable, DSL (uses a phone line but requires some special equipment), and some satellite-based connections are fast and allow lots of information to move rapidly to and from your computer. Dial-up connections are generally slower but cheaper and may be more readily available in some areas. For a dial-up connection you need a regular phone line and a modem (either inside your computer or connected to it), along with an account with an Internet service provider. Most computers today come with a modem as standard equipment (in any case, they are cheap to add) and software already installed to connect you to possible service providers.

You'll need to learn how to open an Internet browser (like Internet Explorer or Firefox in Windows products — the latter is a free open-source download that's my current favorite — or Safari on a Mac computer). A browser lets you access a website or search engine by typing in the address. The "www" you hear about so often is typically the beginning of a website address. It's an acronym for "World Wide Web." For our purposes here, Internet, Web, and Net all refer to the same thing.

A website is a place on the Internet that works a bit like a book. It usually presents you with a list of topics that it focuses on. That list, plus some general information, is typically on the home page. Using the book comparison, the home page is basically like a book's title page and table of contents. Clicking on a topic in the list (using a mouse, or a touch pad on some laptops) takes you to an area where more detailed information about that topic can be found, often including text, audio, pictures, and even movies.

A search engine works a bit like a giant index. You can type in words that describe what you want to know more about and the search engine provides you with a list (often a massive one) of websites that have, or may have, some information about what you're interested in. You can even type questions.

It's worth spending some time learning how to use a search engine properly. Each engine (such as Yahoo.com, Google.com, or Ask.com — there are many others) usually has a tutorial or at least a good explanation of how to get the most out of that particular search engine. Most offer ways to narrow down the number of "hits" (indications of web pages that may have what you're looking for). Being able to focus your search will help you save time and minimize frustration and confusion as you conduct your research.

It will be easy for you to get sidetracked when researching because you'll inevitably come across all sorts of interesting topics that may or may not be relevant to the one you're learning about. It's important for you to stay on track.

If you have the time, however, following interesting topics can be entertaining and informative. It occasionally leads to some surprising and useful stuff. This process led me to a medication I don't think I would have heard about any other way, and after some research I have taken it ever since.

Once you get the hang of moving around on or "surfing" the Net using a search engine, you'll be amazed by what becomes available to you.

RESEARCH AND YOUR SCARY DIAGNOSIS

Your computer and the Internet, used properly, will quickly become invaluable to you when you've been presented with a scary diagnosis.

The first thing to search for on the Net is additional information about your diagnosis — that is, information above and beyond anything given to you by your doctor(s) or the drug companies supplying your medications. Information about drugs, and even about your disease or condition, may come through your doctor or pharmacy but often originates from the pharmaceutical company that patented and produced the drugs applicable to your case.

You need to look for multiple sources of information.

You will come across old information, incomplete information, and just plain bad information.

Once you review some of the top hits produced by your searches, and use a couple of different search engines to ensure a good cross-section of information, you'll quickly get a sense of where you need to go next and what you need to discard.

A massive amount of information will pop up. This is when knowing how to narrow your search, using filters or additional key words to zero in on what you really want to know, will be essential. That may sound confusing or difficult, but as with many things one learns in life, you'll become better and faster at it the more you actually do it. It is easier to do than it is to read about it.

Here's one of the great things about having access to searching the Internet: If you read something you find hard to believe — perhaps like what I said earlier about the number of medical "errors" made each year — a quick search will help you decide. Go ahead, search "errors in medical diagnosis," using any search engine, and see what pops up. I just got 5.5 million hits. Note that "diagnostic errors" is too general as a search phrase. Too much non-medical stuff, such as computer-related information, will pop up.

I have emphasized the importance of verifying information you hear related to your scary diagnosis, regardless of the source. By that I mean don't just accept what you hear from any one doctor or read on any one website as the absolute and only choice or truth. Verification is often as simple as reading several of the "hits" listed when you search something using a search engine. You can also ask your doctor(s) or read books on the subject. If what you find in these ways agrees with the initial information you found, you may choose to move on it. If not, you can type in or ask a question to clarify any inconsistencies you may have come across.

I should note that most newer computers and software enable the computer to read text to you, often including websites. You will have to check that your computer system can support this. Early on

I used this process when "reading" for long periods of time was difficult.

I use the concept of verifying information to encourage you to double- and triple-check things so you can make an educated decision regarding whether the information is believable and useful. Most of the time the Internet is, at the very least, a good starting point for your overall research. And keep in mind that your initial findings on the Net are just that — initial. The Net is excellent for "drilling down" to specifics. Almost anything you come up with will itself contain topics and discussions that should be explored in more detail. I often went to look for and read books that were mentioned as references on websites I visited. Many of those books had lots of details about relatively specific topics.

USER GROUPS

To keep things simple I'd like to call a "user group" any website that allows interactive questions and answers to a group of any kind. This includes forums, online communities, chat rooms, and posting sites. Technical types and purists may question this generalization, but for our purposes, it'll work just fine.

Once you have some idea about some of the treatments you'd like to try, or need more information to help you pin down what you may actually be suffering from, being able to post questions to a related, experienced, and interested group of people can be a tremendous tool.

User groups are typically organized by a general subject, and then by a specific issue within that subject. Many of the large search engines either have their own user groups or can be used to search for them.

To make a reasonably complete search, you may need to try all of the names I noted above — forum, online community, chat room, and posting site.

I particularly like Yahoo's Group section. The current link to this service, as I am writing this, is:

http://health.dir.groups.yahoo.com/dir/Health_Wellness.

And no, I didn't get any encouragement from Yahoo for this plug. I've just found it one of the best sites for this kind of thing.

Most groups are free to join, but you do often need to "register" for them. Some groups attempt to screen participants for a variety of reasons and others don't. Registration is usually about limiting spam (garbage, including sales pitches) and junk emails.

There are all kinds of online groups bringing together all kinds of people to discuss all kinds of issues. Whether it's a hobby, an area of interest, a sport, or a health issue, you'll find a group somewhere on the Internet focused on just about anything you can think of. Yahoo's list is massive.

Many of the conditions or illnesses you may be considering as a potential diagnosis or as alternative diagnoses, or treatment options that grabbed your interest, probably have some kind of group related to them somewhere on the Web.

Most topics will have many related groups, often with slightly different focuses. I started out visiting user groups by identifying ones of interest and reading current and past posts. A post is simply the electronic note — question, answer, or comment — sent in to the site by an individual.

Posting is often done by emailing your post to the user group.

This emailing process is typically built into the site. You don't have to open your email program to use it.

However, because many of these sites work using email directly or indirectly, I highly recommend having more than one email address (most service providers allow you several). Why? Because the email address you use when posting to a group will become available to everyone in that group. Unfortunately, there are always people who will take advantage of this and email you stuff you don't want.

These unsolicited emails may be advertising-related or messages that contain computer viruses. Always use a good virus scanning program and antispyware program on your computer and don't open messages with sender or topic information you don't recognize. Turning off the preview option on many email programs (such as Microsoft Outlook) is probably a good idea as well. The preview mode lets you automatically read part of the email. I read some time back that some computer viruses can infect your computer just by your previewing the email. Apparently you don't have to actually open the email itself for that to happen.

Having several email addresses for different uses will help you identify what is being sent to you and why. It also enables you, if you are receiving too much junk, to abandon the affected email address. If you have extra unused addresses available to you, using different ones for different groups also allows you to narrow down where someone got your address from to begin with.

Posting messages on user groups does not expose you to computer viruses because you are sending and not receiving information. Some of these groups ask if you want to be informed of posts by email. I recommend always saying "no" because you can go to the site and read all the posts you want whenever you like. Automatic emails can cause information overload. The fewer emails sent to you the better when it comes to security and the effective use of your time.

THE BENEFITS OF SHARING INFORMATION

I began by just reading posts as they went up and then searching back to read old posts on specific issues. Many posting sites have some kind of search capability so you can bring up some or all of the posts that mention specific words.

I did this for a couple of weeks when first researching my scary diagnosis. I just read. I just "lurked." It's called lurking because you aren't posting anything yourself so your presence isn't obvious.

It's fine to lurk. Probably the majority of users do just that. But if you have a question, go ahead and ask. A nice part of this process is that many of the members of most groups, at least all the ones I've been exposed to, are well aware of how people new to posting are feeling. They understand that you are unsure and tentative. But they also know you're curious about, and often in need of, the information you're reading about.

Because these user groups are made up mostly of people who have issues in common, it's likely some or all have gone through, or are going through, the same things as you. Many watch for and post the latest relevant news.

These issues include insecurities related to participating in the user group, how to best use the Internet, diagnosis-related concerns, and certainly questions about the things you may want to consider doing to try to help yourself. Groups often discuss their individual experiences with specific treatments and medications, and offer opinions and feedback on how they worked and what side effects were experienced. You may or may not have a similar reaction or result. But knowing how others who have tried a treatment or drug fared gives you valuable information for making fully informed decisions. At the very least, it gives you clues to the right kinds of questions to ask your doctor(s).

I suggest you create and save a little document summarizing your "story." I did this after being asked fairly often for some background about myself, my symptoms, what treatments I had tried, and what drugs or supplements I was taking. You don't need to use your full name (or even your real name for that matter) or include any personal information you may not want the world to see. Never include things like passwords or sensitive information (your social security or social insurance numbers, for example) in posts or emails. You can create your story in any basic word-processing program and cut and paste it into online posts or add to it as needed.

I also often copied and pasted my story (or parts of it) into posts when I was asking a question. This helped give some context to what I was asking and resulted in answers that were more specific and meaningful to me.

You can generally contact any member of a user group directly. Typically the website hosting the group gives you the ability to email someone directly rather than "posting" your message to the group. There are times when this is appropriate and will be productive for everyone involved. But when the group as a whole could benefit from your information or thoughts, it's better for you to post.

Try to avoid user groups that are censored. Monitoring of a group by a moderator can be good, but censoring is a whole different thing. Some of the societies, foundations, associations, and other help groups apparently censor contributions — you can tell by the conspicuous lack of certain information. They often argue that they need to protect the reader. Thanks, but I'd prefer to make up my own mind about what information is useful and what isn't.

It's true that monitoring, which is typically done by the owner of the website, is a sort of partial censorship. But unlike censored sites, properly monitored groups don't restrict information that may represent a contrary or otherwise different opinion. The goal of monitoring should be to keep participants more or less on topic. The specific topic used to identify the group is why most members choose to participate in the group to begin with.

Monitoring should also be used to minimize advertising and soliciting. User groups are easy targets for those trying to expose you to their products, services, or agendas (political, social, or otherwise).

Unfortunately, the temptation to filter information often takes priority when a site is monitored. I believe you and I are capable of making judgments for ourselves on differing, but relevant, opinions. That's why I suggest checking to see whether groups you're considering participating in are monitored, and if so whether the rules governing monitoring are available for review and are reasonable. I often decide not to participate if I believe a group is censored.

I feel the same way about using resources available on some websites. I want the whole story, not just the parts the website owner wants me to hear. So don't get stuck using too few websites too often.

Some members of a group may be lonely or otherwise isolated, or may tend to lose focus, and as a result they discuss all kinds of unrelated issues. This is often referred to as off-topic (OT) chatter. This chatter can be distracting and annoying, but is occasionally interesting and helpful.

If you note this kind of degradation in a group's focus, but you like the group, suggest a secondary group be formed or a chat area be used by those members wanting to discuss unrelated issues. Groups often have chat rooms built into the websites hosting them.

Many groups suggest all off-topic posts start with "OT" in the subject line. If and when chatter becomes too much, you can look for a similar group that stays a bit more focused. You'll be doing a lot of reading, so having everyone stay on topic is a big help.

A last tip is that many of the websites hosting user groups allow users to create new groups. If you find a group is not meeting your needs or you want to focus on something specific, you can start your own group. Typically it's easy and free. If you decide to start and monitor a group, you may be taking on some work, but for some of you, creating and hosting a group may not only yield better results for you but also become something you enjoy doing.

Uncensored user groups, by design, allow for almost anything to be said.

Just because something is posted doesn't mean it's true, complete, or accurate. Sometimes bad information turns up. Occasionally this happens on purpose because someone is using and abusing a good thing for bad reasons.

Often misinformation is posted by well-meaning people who think they're helping.

I've noticed that usually only a small number of users in any given group post regularly. These regular posters are often experienced and knowledgeable. Most of them are genuinely trying to help. Unfortunately, although some regular posters may be knowledgeable on some subjects, they tend to represent themselves as knowledgeable on most subjects. Some posters simply think they know more than they actually do, and some just get confused and don't get the whole story straight.

You need to be cautious, very cautious. Always look to verify the content of any post that interests you.

One of the best things about user groups and the Internet for someone who is ill is also one of the worst things about it — that you and everyone else are anonymous. That's a big plus for an ill person who doesn't want to make his or her illness public knowledge. But how do you know others are who they say they are?

USING INTERNET RESEARCH

Now that you know how to search the Net and the basics about user groups, the next step is to understand all the issues surrounding the disease or condition you've been told you probably have.

At the same time you need to have a close look at deciding for yourself whether you really have what you were diagnosed with or something that can present with similar symptoms but may be something quite different.

What you're trying to do is learn enough to be able to ask specific questions about what's happening to you or even challenge the diagnosis you've received.

You want to get your doctors to confirm your diagnosis as best as possible by considering any and all other options and *eliminating* them.

Take it from someone who's been there. You may think all options were considered thoroughly before you were given your diagnosis, but chances are very good they were not — at least, not as completely and thoroughly as you might like to think.

You don't need to try getting a medical degree online. You do need to get a basic and objective picture of what's going on with you, enabling you to ask questions to help confirm what you've been told, and to help eliminate other possibilities. This often requires learning enough about other potential diagnoses to get your doctor(s) to think about additional tests or the involvement of other doctors.

There are some excellent health and wellness sites on the Internet that may seem like "alternative medicine." (For our purposes here, we'll call "alternative" almost any treatment that is not a prescription medicine or operation.)

Some of these sites often reference articles from medical journals (such as the *Journal of the American Medical Association* and the *New England Journal of Medicine*) and then provide commentary. Of course, if you want you can access many of the sites containing the original articles or studies directly.

I often find sites with this sort of commentary interesting and informative, but that doesn't mean I accept either the article or commentary as necessarily true and accurate (or complete). They are often excellent starting points. I referenced one earlier from Dr. Joseph Mercola at www.mercola.com. There are others, such as Dr. Andrew Weil's at www.drweilselfhealing.com, that, in my opinion, do an excellent job.

Once you feel you've gotten a good general overview, including a good cross-section of opinions on a standard of care or recommended treatment, you are in a position to take a look at any and *all* other options that may be available to you.

These options may include the off-label use of FDA-approved medications, any of many alternative treatments, the use of supplements, the use of food (I don't like using the word "diet"), exercise, and so on.

A brief explanation of off-label use is in order here. Some drugs go through the process of clinical trials and are approved by the FDA in the U.S., or by other governing bodies in other countries, for a very specific condition or disease. This condition or disease is then listed on the label, so to speak. (You may have trouble finding it among all the other stuff.) But many of these drugs end up getting prescribed, and used, for things other than those they were approved for. This happens so often, some estimate the number of total prescriptions written off-label to be somewhere between 23% and 60% of the drugs prescribed in North America. The term "off-label" actually means "for conditions not listed on the label," and such use is very common. Some doctors are open to the idea and do it regularly.

As you continue your research, your list of the potential cures or treatments, above and beyond what are considered standard medical practice, will grow very quickly. They will range from fairly basic and familiar to bizarre and outlandish.

However, remember that what is considered bizarre today may be standard of care tomorrow (or some years from now). When penicillin was discovered it took more than ten years before it was put to regular use. Given that it is derived from mold, one can only imagine what people thought about it back in the 1940s.

Here's another example, from the the introduction to an article about using worms to treat certain diseases.

Doctors at the University of Iowa are testing whether a treatment regimen of worms may help patients with Crohn's disease and ulcerative colitis.

Every three weeks, 15 to 20 patients of Dr. Joel Weinstock and colleagues swallow a mixture of 2,000 eggs of the helminth or parasitic worm, known as porcine whipworm, suspended in Gatorade. Some of them have been on this treatment for more than two years, with excellent results.

"There have been no treatment failures yet and no one has gotten worse," said Weinstock, professor of internal medicine. "The data suggest they seem to get better."

In fact, most of the patients did so well on the therapy they were able to throw away their other drugs, including steroids, which can have serious side effects. The symptoms returned when the patients stopped drinking the mixture ... [10]

Eating worms as medicine? As you search the Internet you need to remain open-minded but very cautious.

If anything catches your eye as a treatment or cure applicable to your case, begin to build a file on it. Here again, a computer is your best tool. You can save Web addresses in your browser by creating file folders, just like paper files stored in a file cabinet (at least in theory). Save any sites you visit that help build or destroy the case for a particular option becoming a viable treatment for you to consider. (This is part of the verification process.) These sites can be saved under Bookmarks, Favorites, or a similar function of your Internet browser.

As you begin to identify potential treatment options, your goal is to eliminate those options as a choice for you. The options that remain form your list of possible treatments you'll likely be choosing from.

This process may be difficult because you will often get conflicting opinions on any given treatment. It's important to remember there are very few absolutes associated with dealing with the kinds of diagnoses we are talking about here. Remember, we rarely know what caused the problem to begin with. Yet some folks, some doctors, some companies, will try to make you believe they know

---

10   Medserv Medical News on the Web at www.medserv.dk

something for sure. I am here to tell you hardly anything is "for sure" when it comes to most scary diagnoses.

This means you need to start playing several roles. Not only are you the detective investigating the case, you are also the lawyers on both sides trying the case, and finally the judge and jury making the decision about whether or not a particular option may be right for you.

AN ONGOING PROCESS

The size of the growing list of potential options may itself become scary.

In all likelihood, whether you know it or not, it took you some time to get really sick. It may therefore take some time to see yourself stabilize and improve. The size of the list should continue to change. New information that becomes available should be added and older information should be confirmed (verified) or discarded.

This, for most of us, will be an ongoing and perhaps never-ending process. It will be never-ending for me unless a "cure" is found for what I have. Even then I think I'll still be double-checking. Since I'm not real sure about what I have, identifying a "cure" may be difficult at best.

You need to remember you're looking for things that may help you. Not just one thing, but almost anything. In most cases there's no magic bullet. Stabilization and recovery will likely include a list of things you'll use short-term, intermittently, or for a long time. If it gets you feeling and getting better, who cares which specific ones worked and why? Often "what works best" is a combination of things. It would be nice to know exactly what worked on what, but rarely can anyone make that connection definitively.

Critics of patients being proactive as opposed to being passive and submissive and critics of anecdotal evidence often point to what I just said as a reason for the patient to take no self-initiated action at all. Leave it to the experts is their position; trial and error is part of the medical process. That confirms, though, that it should also be part of your focus as the patient.

Initially you want to look for things with the best potential results and the least risk. Risk in this case is the potential to have a negative effect on your long-term health and wellness. Even this is tricky, for two reasons: because of the differing opinions on almost any given treatment, and because some treatments actually seem to make you worse initially (or at least you'll *feel* worse initially). They may be addressing some specific problem that your body then needs to cope with. That short-term problem that's being addressed may or may not be directly related to your diagnosis, but it's a problem all the same.

Some of these treatments with what appears at first to be a negative effect or reaction later clear up and have an overall positive effect. This phenomenon seems to be more recognized and accepted among alternative care practitioners but is becoming more accepted among many allopathic doctors (M.D.s) as well. Just not many I've been exposed to.

This initial negative response is often called Herxheimer reaction, or "Herx" for short, by many alternative practitioners. You can enter either term into one of your search engines for lots more information.

NO EASY ANSWERS

You're probably getting a bit frustrated if not downright mad by now. You were no doubt hoping and expecting some kind of easy answer or definite solution. Early on, so was I.

All this computing, reading, sifting, and eliminating takes a lot of work. Searching using a search engine can produce millions of hits. At times it will seem overwhelming, and at times it is. But a scary diagnosis can be even more overwhelming. If something can help you feel better and hopefully get better, or something can improve the quality of your new life, don't you want to know about it? Becoming skilled at narrowing down the number of hits you get when searching is a function of getting to know how to use search engines properly, which comes from experience.

The big surprise for most of us proactive patients is how interesting, compelling, and productive it is to learn, discover, and communicate. The whole process becomes entertaining, fun, and most definitely addictive.

Here's a summary with some helpful hints about being careful as you navigate the Net for answers.

— Initially you just want to better understand what you've been told, and to digest what it really means to you. You need to be extra careful when researching your disease or condition because you will often come across many "worst-case" examples which may *never* have any bearing on your case.
— You can scare yourself sicker. Be careful not to dwell on the worst or extreme cases you may come across in your searching. Always try to assume you have a "mild" case of whatever you've got.
— Be careful with words that get overused and abused, because they start to lose their meaning. These words can represent an important concept, which is often why they get overused to begin with, so make sure you know what they really mean. For example, I came across the words "toxins" and "toxic" so often that they almost shut me down. Unfortunately, words like these are often quite accurate and it's worth getting a good

perspective on the things they refer to and how these may ultimately affect your health.

Searching the Internet can become all-consuming all too quickly. You need to pay attention to things like sleeping, eating properly, and getting a bit of sun and exercise daily if you're going to stabilize and improve your condition. I spent too many late nights searching and thinking, which no doubt delayed my recovery.

Try to stay off the computer before bed. It's tough to shut off your brain, even a foggy one like mine was, right after surfing the Net. Trust me on this one.

SEVEN

NEW PERSPECTIVES ON WELLNESS

And we have made of ourselves living cesspools,
and driven doctors to invent names for our diseases.
— PLATO

I WAS SURPRISED to have more questions *after* my diagnosis than before it. Way more.

I soon realized a diagnosis is a "best guess," there were other conditions that could explain my symptoms, each condition could potentially be addressed by many different treatments, and ... well, let's just say things were getting really complicated.

At the start of this "adventure" I knew only two things for sure. One was that I had better start relying on myself rather than waiting for someone to take me by the hand and get me to my *best* destination. The second was that I hardly knew anything.

My engineering and business backgrounds had taught me that the best way to tackle a problem was to break it down into small pieces and then to put like bits together with like. I knew if I could do that, I would have a fighting chance of piecing together a plan. And, as discussed in the previous chapter, I knew the Internet would prove an excellent research tool for me.

WHAT IS ILLNESS?

Before I could research specific details, I needed to do a reality check on what being sick really meant. I started researching and reading and came to believe there are three basic kinds of illness:

— Everyday illnesses.
— Mechanical illnesses.
— Overload illnesses.

The everyday kind of illness includes conditions like colds and sore throats often blamed on catching some kind of bug.

The mechanical kind includes conditions that can be addressed by an operation to either fix or remove the problem, or by an adjustment by a good chiropractor or osteopath if things get "out of line." Things like tumors, some cancers, and heart disease fit this category of mechanical illnesses — meaning it is at least conceivable an operation will deal with them. But they may also fall into both of the other categories, when you look at why these things may be happening to begin with.

Overload illnesses result from too many problems hitting the patient at once or too many bad things building up in the patient. You may say that "overload" doesn't sound very medical and isn't precise enough because it includes too many variables. But that's precisely my point. I have come to believe the onslaught of stuff that shouldn't be in our bodies is behind many if not most of the health problems we currently face, regardless of which of the two other categories of illness these things may fall into initially.

In fact, I am beginning to think this may be the *only* category of illness.

I believe our bodies are designed to handle pretty much anything we come upon as hunter-gatherers — which is what we were back in the old days before supermarkets, tap water, and processed foods. One of our biggest problems when it comes to staying healthy may be that we no longer need to act like the hunter-gatherers we were designed to be.

OUR IMMUNE SYSTEMS

Humor me for just a moment and picture making tea in a teapot. This analogy will help you see what I mean by our bodies being over-loaded.

First you choose a pot. Teapots come in a variety of shapes and sizes. The spouts are typically even with, or a bit lower than, the opening at the top. This is to allow for easy pouring. To make tea, you pour boiling water into the top opening, having already placed tea leaves (or bags) in the bottom of the pot.

If you're experienced at this, you're careful not to pour too much water in. If you overfill the pot, some of the water or tea is likely to spill out of the spout before you're ready to serve it.

You then let the tea steep, which allows the hot water to become infused by the tea put in the pot. The longer you do this, the stronger the brew.

Now you can serve the tea.

When the teapot is well designed, and the tea is prepared and served properly, nothing is spilled and the tea is just right. If not — for instance, if there is a design weakness in the teapot or too much water is added — the tea will spill before you're ready to pour.

If you let the tea steep too long it becomes way too strong and tastes terrible.

Now *really* humor me and picture people, or more specifically their immune systems, as teapots.

Like teapots, we come in a variety of sizes and shapes. Some of us have differently shaped spouts located in different places. These spouts and their locations are the result of our genetic predispositions to certain illnesses or diseases.

Picture a genetic predisposition as a weak spot, the place the tea will pour out of first because the spout is "designed" to work that way.

In everyday life we expose ourselves to all kinds of things that can make us sick. These potentially bad things are in the air, water, and food, in or on other people, and possibly in or on our pets. They can also originate in our minds and be self-inflicted, at least in part — sometimes as a result of stress or an emotional reaction or mental response or condition.

When our bodies are healthy and our organs are functioning correctly, we can fight off most of this stuff effortlessly. The bad stuff we're exposed to is like the water and tea put into the teapot. Nothing spills out — the pot can hold what's being put into it.

If you're living with wellness in mind, you're careful about what you breathe, drink, and eat, and you get lots of rest and exercise. You're careful about what you put into your pot. It takes a long time, maybe your whole life, to fill the pot. By being careful you also prevent your "tea" from steeping too much and becoming too strong.

Part of being careful is to avoid thinking yourself into a state of tension and stress.

You can essentially turn off the tap that's filling the pot by being careful. Or at least you can cut down how fast you're "filling up." Being careful and aware can prevent your pot from filling up and prematurely pouring out of your spout and making a mess.

If you're actively working on wellness, you may actually be emptying out some of the tea in your pot, slowly and carefully and in a controlled fashion. This prevents the pot from overflowing, and allows more stuff to be added to the pot without the tea getting too strong or the pot too full.

This emptying-out process is often called "detoxing." Your body does some of this naturally through bathroom visits, breathing, sweating, and other means. Some people work at helping their bodies eliminate some of the bad stuff that tends to accumulate. This is often done by "cleanses," fasting, or enemas and colonics.

Cleanses rely on formulas (usually herbal with some supplements) and specific foods and drinks to help your body release and eliminate bad stuff.

Fasting takes the pressure off your body of processing and eliminating new food, allowing it to eliminate old stuff, although most fasts include lots of specific fluids.

Colonics are basically super-enemas, administered by another person (enemas can be self-administered) using appropriate equipment that essentially washes your insides, loosening old material from your bowels, allowing them to get cleaner than they typically do. In general, the cleaner your bowels, the better they work to remove and eliminate waste from your body.

People often use combinations of these techniques to get the best results. As usual, the key is to get the best results for you given your current condition.

Most of us don't live this way. We aren't careful or conscious and don't pay attention as our pot starts to fill up or the "tea" gets too strong, little by little, every day.

Sometimes, depending on how you live and what you're exposed to, your pot fills up surprisingly fast. This can happen to kids because of their small size and lack of wellness skills. What they are encouraged to eat and drink (refined white sugar, artificial sweeteners, and processed foods being prime examples) can overload them much too quickly. There are also some serious and growing questions about some medications and vaccinations administered to kids.

Now remember, the tea is like the bad stuff taxing your immune system. The more it builds up, the less room there is for new stuff to fit into the pot, and the stronger the tea.

The same thing happens to your body and immune system. As the bad stuff builds, spillage becomes inevitable.

Now what about the matter of genetic predisposition? Well, that means we have a weakness passed on from our parents. That's right; we may be able to blame our parents, at least a little, when we hear our scary diagnosis. If genetic predispositions usually vary from person to person, they can be very similar in the case of blood relatives. Some diseases or conditions are said to run in the family, putting you and your blood relatives at risk for similar health problems.

Remember, such a predisposition is like the spout on the teapot. If we have some kind of genetic weak spot, the tea will begin spilling out through this spot as our immune system is overwhelmed.

We end up getting symptoms or conditions based on how big our spouts are, where they happen to be located, and what went into our tea to begin with, along with how strong we allowed the brew to get.

Similar teapots or similar brews may mean similar illnesses and diagnoses. But unless each teapot is almost the same and filling up at nearly the same time and with a similar brew, one person may show symptoms while another does not. These days all of us get exposed to lots of the same things. It may be at different times and in different amounts, but our constantly shrinking world means very similar bad stuff is eventually reaching most of us.

Some of us get "sick" while others don't. Unless your pot is almost full, it probably won't start spilling over because the critical level dictated by your exposure, your focus on wellness, and your very own genetic predisposition has not been reached. Your diagnosis will depend not only on the size and shape of your pot but on what you put into it.

You can see, based on all this, that you have some control.

Remember, the pot gets filled a bit at a time. Over time you're left with a blend of bad stuff that has accumulated from air, water, food, chemicals and bugs of various sizes and shapes, topped off by a nice measure of stress. Stress (an issue we'll discuss in more detail in chapter eleven) is like stirring in acid or sugar.

All the things that went into creating your brew, including the pot, are factors combining to produce the finished products. Those products are your symptoms and they are eventually given a name by a doctor.

That's right. Your very own scary diagnosis.

Since we have some control over what we put into our bodies, let's talk a bit about "being careful" with what we expose our bodies to. Being careful and aware of what we eat and drink is a good preventative move. It's also a good maintenance or treatment move *after* you become ill.

WELLNESS

Regardless of what anyone says, being consciously aware of wellness is important. Here's a quick definition from Answers.com:

> **well·ness (w_l'n_s) n.**
> The condition of good physical and mental health, especially when maintained by proper diet, exercise, and habits.[11]

What we eat, drink, breathe, and think are pieces of most illness puzzles. All too often they don't receive the "credit" they deserve. If we pay attention to exposing ourselves to things that are right for our individual bodies and limiting exposure to things that are wrong for them, we should be able to keep remarkably healthy simply through regular maintenance.

I can't help but wonder how many of our health problems would disappear if we (society, business, and the world in general) understood and prioritized "wellness" — if we made a plan to achieve and maintain health and implemented it. Wellness is all about protecting ourselves from allowing our bodies, minds, and immune systems from becoming overwhelmed and overflowing.

This requires two kinds of action. The first is minimizing exposure to things that can accumulate in us and make us sick sooner or later. The second involves doing things to help keep our bodies, minds, and immune systems from getting overloaded. Let's look at each of these in turn.

---

11 http://www.answers.com/topic/wellness

Minimizing Exposure

We need to be careful about what we breathe, drink, eat, think, and do. Lots of things need watching and some are as familiar as the foods we eat every day. Food may either contain bad stuff, or, for several different reasons, not be seen as "good" by our individual bodies — even though you may have been told this food was good for you since you were a child.

What is "good" for some bodies may be bad for others. Your genetic predisposition may play a role in this as well.

The main message of this book is to be proactive and take control of your own health and life. A great way to make a start at this is to learn about what to eat and drink, how to exercise and live, and how to reduce stress.

We don't like to hear it, but it's true: Almost everything we do has a consequence.

We certainly don't want to hear the ever more common message that almost everything we eat, drink, breathe, or touch may be bad for us. Our homes, our cars, our schools, and our workplaces and the environmental issues associated with them may have a serious impact on our health. We can actually be poisoning ourselves slowly just by living our regular lives. Chances are pretty good this is exactly what's happening to most of us.

A great example of this was in the news recently.

The prime minister of Canada announced a new policy cracking down on chemicals affecting consumers:

> The new strategy "will make Canada a world leader in testing and regulation of chemicals that are used in thousands of consumer products."

Although the preliminary review by scientists at Health
Canada and Environment Canada has found that thousands
of chemicals pose hazards, the government will focus on the
500 most dangerous ...[12]

So what are all these bad things that we are exposed to every day?
They can be the paint on the walls, the chemicals in the carpet or
fabric, the cleaning products we use (or that are used by someone
else), poor air quality, inappropriate kind of light, the auto fumes in
the garage attached to our houses or that we breathe as we drive.
Well, you get the idea.

We put all kinds of things on our skin and hair. Ever read the
labels on those bottles? Our skin provides a huge surface area that's
good at absorbing things. In a shower the warm water opens our
pores, enhancing absorption even more. Be careful what you use in
the shower. For instance, when you wash your hair, the shampoo
runs down over your entire body. The stuff in some shampoos may
be okay for hair, but how about for the rest of you, especially inside
you? Have a good look at the ingredients and do a little research.
Lotions and perfumes are absorbed or inhaled, so have an extra good
look at those.

Underarm deodorants need to be carefully scrutinized and used
(especially if you're ill), because they typically contain metals like
aluminum and other potentially harmful ingredients. The area under
our arms is a prime area for maximum absorption. Unfortunately,
many of the more natural products currently available don't perform
as well as we may be used to. We as a society may need to reconsider
what we find acceptable with respect to the performance of many of
the products we currently use and take for granted.

This is important stuff whether you're sick or not.

---

12   The *Globe and Mail*, December 9, 2006, p. A1.

Some people are tuned into these environmental health issues without getting the wake-up call of getting sick. Others don't stop and take a good look at these things until they're very ill. Some people choose, for various reasons, to ignore or reject potential problems. That's a very big mistake.

It's more than just the obvious or "popular" stuff like fungus (mold), viruses, and bacteria that we need to be on the lookout for. In the world we live in it's *everything everywhere*, unless you live in a pristine place where there's no pollution (little to no industry), you can drink the water directly out of a stream (please don't unless you're sure), and everything you build with, eat, drink, put on or in your body, and wear is natural and chemical-free.

I'm guessing that no one reading this lives in such a place. There may not be any left. You'd think maybe the North and South Poles would qualify, but planes fly over these spots, and electromagnetic waves and fallout from nuclear testing and accidents show up there, too.

When we're healthy it makes sense that most of us (except for an enlightened few) spend little or no time thinking about these things. We don't have the time and quite frankly it just isn't real enough to us to be an issue in our daily lives. It's easier not to add to the stress and disrupt our busy routines. It's easier to make light of, or even fun of, this stuff.

But then when were not so healthy, some of us start wondering, why us?

Once you begin to look for answers it seems almost everything can have some kind of impact on your health. Most of the time the potential impact of our personal environment seems more negative than positive. That really gets some people thinking — and has other people shutting down.

Right about now you may be thinking, "Enough bad news, thank you."

It's confusing and frustrating, but when you're focused on wellness or you're ill, it may be critically important for you to be aware of your own environment. If you pay close attention your body may actually tell you what's good and bad for it.

The old cliché "you are what you eat" is only part of the story. In today's world, you are what you eat, drink, breathe, think, and put on your hair and skin and into your mouth. How your body processes and eliminates all of the above is also part of what you are.

Preventing Overloading

The next move, after minimizing your exposure to potentially harmful things, is to actually prevent your immune system from getting overloaded in the first place. One way to do this is to keep your body fit and well-maintained. This includes keeping things flowing properly. Proper elimination and drinking plenty of good water are key.

In addition, you should occasionally flush out your system. As described above, purposeful detoxing or cleansing is like giving your insides a bath. You're essentially just cleaning things out and letting them flow down the drain. Sometimes a detox program is called a cleanse. Detoxification can be summed up by saying that you do thngs to pour out or dilute some of your "tea." If you don't deal with the buildup of "tea" or bad stuff, illness is often the result.

The symptoms of illness often include ways of eliminating some of the bad stuff implicated in the illness. Vomiting, diarrhea, fevers, and skin rashes or breakouts are just a few of the ways our bodies try to get rid of something bad.

Many of us understand the value of maintaining our vehicles

more than we understand the value of maintaining our bodies. Regular service, changing the oil, flushing out the radiator, and rotating the tires are preventative measures and are designed to keep our vehicles running smoothly and safely. Perhaps we're better at maintaining our vehicles because most of us pay someone else to actually do the work.

That doesn't really work with wellness. Wellness requires active participation. It requires some education, because most of us seem somewhat mystified about our bodies, including me.

The truth is, many health issues start with the basics, and these basics are really basic. A big problem these days seems to be the huge difference of opinion about what the basics actually are. Prioritizing them can change dramatically from source to source and even from day to day. One day coffee is good for you, and the next day someone is screaming, "Don't drink that poison!" Who's right and when? By now you probably know the answer — that there is no easy answer. But you can increase your chances of making good choices by taking control and being proactive. Make educated decisions and apply some common sense. It's a question of making and keeping health and wellness a top priority.

EXTENDING THE FAMILY OF AUTOIMMUNE DISEASES

In terms of the history of medicine, the autoimmune diseases seem relatively "new." Although theories abound as to what causes them, they seem to fit my teapot analogy nicely.

Some of the symptoms are quite similar from one autoimmune disease to another. Many autoimmune diseases have such long lists of possible symptoms, the names or labels given to these diseases or conditions are almost (and occasionally are) interchangeable.

If you've been told you have an autoimmune condition (such as MS), that diagnosis is often based on your symptoms or on very general clues such as test results, which only offer indicators rather than something definitive.

Doctors may resist extending the label of autoimmune diseases to other conditions thought to be caused in other ways. However, medical researchers are beginning to test medications and treatments for some autoimmune conditions on other autoimmune conditions. For example, "Taking a drug used for Alzheimer's disease may improve the memory of people with multiple sclerosis, according to a study published in the November 9, 2004, issue of *Neurology*, the scientific journal of the American Academy of Neurology."[13]

And they're testing non-autoimmune treatments on autoimmune diseases. For example, "A cancer chemotherapy drug is the first effective treatment for certain forms of advanced multiple sclerosis and should be approved today by a panel of scientific experts from the Food and Drug Administration."[14]

What about cancer? Talking about all cancers at once doesn't make much sense. Some are quite different from others. But I believe some are at least partially the result of an overtaxed and overwhelmed immune system.

Sometimes cancer can be very specific, attacking an organ that may be a weak spot in a person's health, perhaps as the result of a genetic predisposition. Other cancers are more systemic, traveling through the fluid-carrying systems of blood or lymph.

How different is cancer from autoimmune conditions? Is an MS patient's myelin being sick or dying that much different from a

---

13   http://www.sciencedaily.com/releases/2004/11/041123114858.htm
14   http://query.nytimes.com/gst/fullpage.html?sec=health&res=9F03#4D7113
      CF93AA15752C0A9669C8B63

cancer patient's cells becoming cancerous? Are the mechanisms somehow similar? Are the triggers or root causes related?

These questions currently have no definitive answers.

What about the cardiovasucular system? Circulation problems and heart issues are often referred to as "plumbing." In a building, most plumbing problems are first addressed by applying a plunger or drain cleaner before a snake is used or pipes are replaced. Yet if we're careful with what we dump down the drain to begin with, and occasionally use a bit of drain cleaner to keep things running smoothly, snaking or replacing pipes becomes the exception and not the rule.

Heart and circulation issues must be related, at least in part, to what we eat, drink, and breathe. How we live (lifestyle) and what we're exposed to daily contributes at least in some way to most health issues.

Stress

The word "stress" can mean different things. It comes in lots of flavors. You can stress your body through exercise or lack of it; by exposing yourself to a harmful environment containing fumes, bacteria, fungus, etc. (which unfortunately can include your home, car, and place of work); or by fixating negatively on an issue.

When we refer to stress we are typically talking about the kind that comes from emotional or mental fixations. What we think and feel clearly affects us physically. If you doubt this, do a bit of research on how what we think can have measurable results on our bodily functions. Worry is stress and stress causes worry. It's a vicious circle.

Our health and wellness is related to whether we're being overwhelmed with things that are bad for us. And guess what's right in there pitching when it comes to things that are bad for us? Stress.

Nowadays even kids are overstressed by school and extracurricular activities, as well as by situations at home.

A scary diagnosis only makes things worse. Indecision causes stress. So does the fact that we know so little about so many conditions, and that drugs are typically symptom-focused rather than cure-focused.

How we think creates or intensifies our bodies' reactions. I have no doubt that regardless of whatever viruses, bacteria, fungi, parasites, or toxic load may have caused or triggered my condition, the way I was handling stress was a contributing factor.

In other words, I played an active role in causing some of the symptoms that prompted my scary diagnosis.

Stress is no doubt a contributing factor to almost any scary diagnosis, whether we currently understand how or not.

The next time you're stressing out over something trivial — like someone cutting you off in traffic — think about what you're doing to yourself and what you may be triggering.

Nutrition and Digestion

Food and nutrition are major issues and they will be covered in detail in chapter eleven. But it's worth touching on digestion here.

I believe "we are what we digest, absorb, and utilize" is a much more accurate statement when it comes to food than "we are what we eat."

When I began reading about MS and all the other things I might possibly have, I was shocked by how digestion-related issues kept popping up everywhere — except in the offices and examining rooms of doctors and specialists.

I noted that a fairly large number of MS patients conversing on user groups mentioned bad digestion. Just as an additional point of interest, sinus problems were also common. In fact, there are some interesting discussions as to whether and how digestion and sinus issues may be related. I myself had been having "stomach problems" prior to the attack of optical neuritis leading to my MS diagnosis. And I have had sinus problems since forever.

I decided to do some searches on the Internet and I again found poor digestion mentioned as a possible factor in all kinds of health issues, not just MS.

I began to think a lot about digestion. I thought about all the commercials I had seen for various stomach medications: pills for acid, pills for diarrhea, pills for gas, and pills for bloating (which generally involves gas).

All of a sudden it made perfect sense to me.

What if I wasn't digesting food and vitamins properly, even if they were the right food and supplement choices for me (which they probably weren't)? How could I possibly be getting many of the basic things my body needed in order to be healthy?

But why was my digestion so bad? Why is it that most people's digestion is so bad, or at the very least up and down?

After all, the commercials are aired because lots of people are suffering from digestion problems. But are these drugs and over-the-counter medications fixing the problems, or just endlessly dealing with symptoms? In our world of modern conveniences and modern medicine, why are so many people experiencing these problems to begin with?

Perhaps I was to blame for my bad digestion. Was my choice of foods and supplements somehow affecting my digestion? Was my choice of beverages and when I drank them somehow an issue? Was stress the culprit?

Now that I was ill, I not only needed to understand my condition by researching and questioning my diagnosis, I also needed to understand how to get the most benefit out of what went into my body. I'm talking about food, liquid, and air — the basics of life.

Were my choices causing my digestion problems, or was poor digestion a symptom of my MS diagnosis or something else entirely?

I began to wonder if the large assortment of antibiotics and other drugs I had taken over the years were part of the problem. I'm not saying I should or shouldn't have taken any or all of these drugs. I'm simply wondering whether they had a cumulative effect on me, and more specifically on my digestion. After all, have you ever listened to the disclaimers that are pretty much part of every over-the-counter and prescription drug commercial on television and radio? Have you ever read the fine print listing the side effects of any of the drugs you may be taking? Have you ever wondered, if you're taking several drugs, how each one may be affecting the others and how, together, they are affecting you?

I was growing more concerned with how to fix my digestion problems because I had mentioned them to all the doctors I had seen after day one of fuzzy eye (and for years off and on before that) and not one thought these problems were important with respect to my MS symptoms.

I felt I had to get my system functioning, because without proper digestion how could I hope to feel better day to day and even meal to meal?

I had lost almost 22 pounds in three months since my diagnosis. Not good for someone 5 feet 11 inches tall who had weighed 172 pounds for as long as he could remember. At 150 pounds I didn't feel healthy and although I didn't realize it, I certainly didn't look healthy, either.

If I didn't start to feel better, how could I tolerate additional medication, knowing that many warn of side effects involving the stomach, liver, and kidneys?

I wasn't sure what the various organs of my body actually did and what impact, if any, they had on digestion. But my gut, literally and figuratively, was telling me this was important.

If you aren't eliminating properly, is it a good idea to have any number of drugs interacting with any number of chemicals from food, drink, and general exposure sitting for extra long periods of time in your gut? Do the drugs you take list "constipation" as a potential side effect?

What about drugs designed to be "digested" in order to be absorbed and work properly?

As a starting point, ask your doctor about your digestion and elimination, and how they may relate to your scary diagnosis. Stick with it to get good, clear answers. Digestion, regardless of whether it contributes to your symptoms or is inhibited by them, is a very big deal. Regardless of what anyone else tells you, be sure to research this subject for yourself.

EIGHT

ALTERNATIVE MEDICINE
AND THE FUTURE OF MEDICINE

We must admit that we have never fought the homeopath
on matters of principle. We fought them because they
came into our community and got the business.
— DR. J.N. McCORMACK

ONE OF THE steps in your action plan is searching for information
on your condition. Not long after you start doing this, you're going
to come across all kinds of health and treatment options.

You may be suspicious of some of the options because you've
never heard of them before. You may dismiss some of them because
they don't seem relevant to you and your condition.

Other options you may find more challenging, because they
bring into question things you've been told, often by doctors and
other healthcare professionals. You may learn that some of the foods,
treatments, and procedures you consider safe are in fact potentially
harmful to you.

Asking questions about health and wellness, reading, researching, and applying some common sense may well turn your everyday world upside down. It did for me.

This chapter discusses some of these remedies, treatments, issues, and opinions under the topic of alternative medicine and the future of medicine.

A WORLD OF POSSIBILITIES

Some of the old-time remedies, including topical treatments (lotions, salves, and poultices), tonics, elixirs and other drinkables (potions), a huge variety of teas (herbal and otherwise), and things as offbeat as bee stings and as commonplace as honey can all play a role in alternative medicine.

Some really basic things work remarkably well in addressing some issues. Enzymes are a good example. You can take them with food to aid digestion. You can take them without food to help reduce inflammation (wherever it may be occurring). This harks back to times when enzymes were more plentiful in our diets. I find the product Wobenzymes®, when taken with lots of water on an empty stomach, is useful as a pain reliever. I haven't taken an aspirin, Tylenol, Advil, or the like for years.

You may be surprised by what you find if you take the time to look up "side effects" or "interactions" for everyday, over-the-counter pain relievers. Do an Internet search of acetylsalicylic acid (aspirin), ibuprofen (like Advil®), and other painkillers. You'll see arguments that some of these things have negative effects, especially long-term.

Enzymes and probiotics help digestive problems. Do the same Internet search for some of the stomach-related over-the-counter drugs as well.

People think side effects and interactions affect only a small percentage of the population adversely, but after receiving a scary diagnosis, chances are you're now part of that small percentage. It's worth noting that many of us experience minor side effects we've been trained to, or choose to, ignore. Choosing to ignore them is usually a function of getting short-term results for a specific symptom without understanding or recognizing long-term effects on our overall health. The training part relates to the constant barrage of marketing material and sales pitches that shift our attention from potential side effects, especially "minor" ones. But who decides what's minor and over what time frame?

Some herbal teas work well on a variety of things. Eating the right foods — where "right" means the foods that are right for you as opposed to the latest wonder diet (for health or weight loss) — can work wonders. I find chamomile tea soothes my stomach. A doctor recommended I drink licorice root tea when my blood pressure was consistently low, and it worked great over the course of several weeks. Although I love ice cream, my digestive system doesn't. I find this true of most dairy products. They seem to make my sinuses stuff up or run as well.

MSG (Monosodium glutamate) is a food additive, marketed as a flavor enhancer, that makes me numb in my face and knees. It is often found in Chinese food and in lots of canned products like soup. I can always "feel" when something has a bunch of MSG in it. Yet when I eat a meal of fish, vegetables, and some rice or steak and veggies (no starch), I generally feel great with no signs of stomach distress. You may find these combinations aren't for you. You should experiment a bit to find what works best for your system.

COMPOUNDING PHARMACIES

Sometimes your options are more mainstream but not particularly well-known. Take compounding pharmacies, for example. These specialty pharmacies, at your doctor's instruction, can prepare doses that are lower or higher than the standard pill size. The size of the minimum dose set by regular pharmacies is based on averages. That means you may find that the lowest dose you can get for a drug is 10 mg, though in your case 5 mg may yield the same or more acceptable results. You may be taking a pill that would work better or help you feel better if the dose or filler is changed.

Some fillers used in pills and capsules are made of substances that may affect patients adversely. For example, corn products are often used. This means patients allergic to corn probably shouldn't take drugs containing such fillers.

Many drugs can be prepared in forms that make them easier to use. These include lotions, creams, liquids, and patches for topical applications. These applications can be adjusted to make drugs more acceptable to the body by eliminating the shock and discomfort of an injection or eliminating the problem some folks have with swallowing pills. I was able to switch from a hormone injection to a cream, which seemed to work better — and with no needle!

Through compounding pharmacies, you can get custom-filled prescriptions using doses and fillers that are best for you. These pharmacies are more numerous than you may think. If there isn't one near where you live, search the Internet for the many that will ship customized prescriptions right to your door.

Think of what you get at these pharmacies as "custom" drugs (as opposed to designer drugs, which have a whole different meaning).

WHAT'S OLD IS NEW: COLLOIDAL SILVER

Just because something is old doesn't mean it has no value today.

Consider, for example, colloidal silver (CS). In the past, tiny particles of silver were dissolved in a liquid as a sort of a pre-antibiotic antibiotic. And apparently some farmers used to put a silver coin (back when they were really silver) into the milking bucket to keep milk fresher longer. Some hospitals still use CS to clear newborns' eyes. It's also used on bandages for burns and more recently on bandages for cuts and scrapes.

CS is available in most health food stores. Search the Internet for information on it. You'll get a huge number of hits.

Some of those hits are people spreading the good news (old news) about using CS to cure or treat a variety of things from sinus infections to MS and AIDS. Others are selling it. Many claim it is not only an antibiotic but also an antifungal and antiviral.

As an alternative medicine it is also often recommended as one of the more effective yeast infection treatments for women, as featured on the television show *The View* (Friday, October 9, 2006).

As with pretty much anything, there are potential downsides to CS. In your research you'll come across the warning it will turn you blue if you take too much of it. This is called agryria and is caused by impure CS or by taking too much of it (there are differing opinions on the right amounts). Turning blue is extremely rare, requiring consumption of a large amount internally over a long time, or it may be related to the type or quality of CS. People negative about CS, and some who sell it, make it sound like you'll be blue tomorrow, or that everyone will turn blue if it's used at all or unless their brand is used.

Others claim it never happens. I believe it does, but very rarely.

I came across CS when researching MS. I found some MSers claimed it "cured" their condition. My guess is for some it did — or at least it helped control their symptoms and the progression of the disease. I don't doubt that some saw their symptoms disappear if their MS had a bacterial or possibly fungal or viral trigger and CS reduced or eliminated those triggers. Others have tried it with no major effect.

Perhaps the successes were in people who were misdiagnosed. Not all Lyme disease patients achieve major results from CS, even though this disease is thought to be a bacterial infection. But there is statistical evidence that some MSers may actually have Lyme, which is treatable (especially early on) with antibiotics.

I believe successful treatments and "cures" do happen, and they happen for a reason. I've used colloidal silver in a nose spray for more than a year now. I am not blue, literally or figuratively. My sinuses are consistently clearer than ever before. It took some time, but they are continuing to improve.

The first sprays burned a bit, but that only convinced me the treatment was doing something the antibiotics and sprayed steroids I used before had failed to do.

Was this a coincidence of some kind? Perhaps.

Although I'd like to know for certain whether CS is responsible for my improvement, I know from my experience as a test engineer it's very difficult to isolate the performance of a single thing being added to a complex system. I made lots of changes in lifestyle and diet at more or less the same time, so it's hard to credit CS alone.

The human body is complex to begin with. There's much we still don't know about how and why it functions the way it does. Adding to that complexity and uncertainty the conditions that resulted in a scary diagnosis often makes it very challenging to isolate the performance of *anything* given to address either symptoms or causes. This is certainly something to consider when contemplating how much weight to give the findings of a clinical trial.

So while we may not completely understand why cs works, that's nothing new. We routinely use a prescription or over-the-counter drug when we aren't sure what caused the disease it's treating or why the drug seems to work. Most of us don't really understand how most things work, like cell phones or microwave ovens. Why, then, do we treat an alternative medicine with such skepticism when we know it helps (at the very least some people, at a rate not unlike the statistical performance of some drugs) but don't know why?

HORMONES

Other things you should be considering are deemed to be mainstream by some and alternative by others. Hormones, for example.

I first came across this topic when researching ms and autoimmune conditions in general. I read in several places that women with ms, sometimes severe ms, often went into remission when pregnant. It was assumed the hormonal changes related to pregnancy had something to do with these remissions.

That got me thinking and reading more about hormones in general. As a point of reference, here's a brief definition:

Hormones
Chemical substances having a specific regulatory effect on the activity of a certain organ or organs. The term was originally applied to substances secreted by various endocrine glands

and transported in the bloodstream to the target organs. It is sometimes extended to include those substances that are not produced by the endocrine glands but that have similar effects.[15]

Searching the Internet revealed there were all kinds of people thinking about hormones and their link to health and wellness. Some were focused on staying healthy while others were more focused on staying or feeling younger.

Do your own research on this subject, particularly if you're 30 or older. Anyone with an autoimmune issue should spend a bit of time on it. When I told my wife I was researching hormones, she suggested I read a book by Suzanne Somers: *The Sexy Years: Discover the Hormone Connection — The Secret to Fabulous Sex, Great Health, and Vitality, for Women and Men*. Somers, in my opinion, not only does a great job of summarizing information I had read in a variety of places but also touches on some interesting stuff in general. She recommends people get a baseline when they're younger so that know what "normal" is for them (a point I loved as an engineer). In addition, she gets into the importance of bioidentical versus synthetic hormone treatments. It is well worth noting that she's also a cancer survivor.

I went to my out-of-the-box doc (more on this later in this chapter) and asked about hormones and hormone-replacement therapy. At the time he felt it was a low-priority item, but something to watch. I kept bugging him because I had read enough to make me think hormone supplementation could help me.

He had tested me for my testosterone level and I was in the "normal" range.

After I pestered him for several months, he met with me to discuss this. He said he'd just returned from a conference on autoimmune issues. One entire afternoon had been dedicated to hormones.

We discussed my previous tests and had a new test done. I was testing "normal," but for me that meant 4.3 in a range of 4–12. I was within the normal range, but just barely. The information at the conference had indicated autoimmune patients did better at the higher end of the range.

I had my first injection of testosterone that day.

The very next day I felt "better." I was hitting golf balls on a practice range and it felt like my balance was a bit better and I had steadier eye-hand coordination.

Yes, it could have been a coincidence or "just in my head" — except I continued to improve. By "improve" I mean I felt better in subtle ways. Last time I was tested for testosterone I was 11.5, toward the upper end of the "normal" range. (Please note: I believe the scale I referred to has been replaced with a new one. These numbers may not be in sync with the new system of measuring.)

People these days are living longer, whether they are healthy or not. It makes sense to me that hormones should be a relevant topic to many of us. As we get older we seem to naturally produce fewer hormones. I also think the teapot analogy applies here. As we fill up with junk and marinate in that junk, we produce fewer hormones than normal, or the hormones we do produce have little chance of doing what they are supposed to do.

Some may argue hormones are a mainstream, or allopathic, issue. Others would agree they are pretty much a gray area. I think they're important and both women and men should have their hormones tested. It really is a great idea to baseline your "normal levels" when you are younger and healthier because "normal" may not tell you what you really need to know.

To this day I supplement with testosterone. I've switched to a topical cream, thanks to those fabulous compounding pharmacies I told you about. I believe the cream works better because I get a small dose daily (lately every other day). And it's great I don't have to go in for, and endure, the shots.

ELIMINATION

Elimination may be addressed by both mainstream and alternative practitioners (specifically those doing colonics).

The fact is, most of us are marinating our insides in a toxic or otherwise unclean environment. This may be a huge problem affecting all aspects of our health.

If waste is getting "stuck" inside our systems, our bodies are basically swimming in waste, and waste is, by definition (at least in my book), bad.

It's bad and toxic and taxes almost every organ and cell in your body one way or another. Even if you're eating lots of fruits and vegetables, avoiding refined wheat and sugar, drinking lots of water, taking supplements, and on and on, there is no way you're getting the maximum benefits from all this if you aren't eliminating properly. If you are actually doing these things, your elimination should be improving, but research confirms that sometimes, after years of abusing ourselves, we still need some extra help.

All kinds of flushes and cleanses are available to help with this. Fiber is another big subject worth researching. Although they seem a bit weird to most at first, enemas and colonics are good ways to help move things along more easily and naturally.

Taking laxatives or any additional medication just isn't what you want to do if you're ill, though this is often the allopathic approach. There are some more natural things you can take, such as castor oil, but they should be viewed as short-term solutions. You want to be addressing the reason you need a laxative if you have an ongoing problem, instead of just focusing on the symptom.

Enemas have been around for a very long time and were often considered the first line of defense in maintaining health and dealing with illness. Modern medicine seems to have pushed them to the side in favor of laxatives and drugs, but this is one old-time remedy I believe we can all benefit from.

Take a serious look at enemas and colonics (which are "super-enemas"). Regardless of your health, consider giving them a try. If you are ill in any way, enemas should be high on your list of possible treatments.

BACTERIA

A large part of digestion happens with the help of bacteria. We have some good bacteria that helps us process food and some bad bacteria that can be harmful to us. This is from the Mayo Clinic website:

Lactobacilli are bacteria that normally live in the human small intestine and vagina. *Lactobacillus acidophilus* is generally considered to be beneficial because it produces vitamin K, lactase, and anti-microbial substances such as acidolin, acidolphilin, lactocidin, and bacteriocin. Multiple human trials report benefits of *L. acidophilus* for bacterial vaginosis. Other medicinal uses of *L. acidophilus* are not sufficiently studied to form clear conclusions.

The term "probiotic" is used to describe organisms that are

used medicinally, including bacteria such as *L. acidophilus* and yeast such as *Saccharomyces boulardii*.[16]

Foods and beverages, lifestyle and medications can have an impact on the balance of good and bad bacteria in our bodies. Your pH level (the acidity of your bodily fluids — most of us are too acidic) and antibiotics can be key issues. Antibiotics kill bacteria but typically can't tell which bacteria are good and which aren't.

Of course you need to check all this out with your doctor or pharmacist, but most will tell you there is only an upside to adding probiotics to your diet. It amazes me that it has yet to become standard of care to prescribe or at least suggest taking a probiotic after a course of antibiotics, but time will no doubt fix that.

OUT-OF-THE-BOX DOCS AND CHELATION THERAPY

Let's have a look at medical doctors who — some would claim, anyway — are bit more on the "fringe." For the sake of simplicity let's refer to these non-mainstream doctors as out-of-the-box docs (box docs for short).

Some of these box docs have become convinced, for one reason or another, that things like intravenous chelation therapy, high dosages of vitamin C, bioidentical hormone replacement therapy, intravenous hydrogen peroxide, and any of a host of other treatments are sometimes worthy treatment options. Typically they supplement these options with vitamins and minerals along with conventional prescription drugs.

These may or may not be accepted as viable treatments by mainstream doctors or specialists or those trained in integrative medicine. (The integrative type of medical practice will be defined

16 http://www.mayoclinic.com/health/lactobacillus/NS_patient-acidophilus

later in this chapter.) They may be treatments that, although most would consider them alternative, require a doctor to administer.

Based on results reported directly to me in conversations with some patients, some of these treatments have sometimes been as effective as, more effective than, and occasionally far more effective than the standard of care for their condition. I have come to believe they are definitely worth a look for cancer, heart and circulation, and autoimmune conditions — and that they also show some real promise for autism.

Intravenous chelation for heart and circulatory issues has often been a choice of last resort for patients who have reached the end of their options or who have been sent home by those offering more conventional treatments. Many of these applications are currently considered an off-label use of chelation, given that it is the standard of care for lead and mercury poisoning.

Sadly, there is little accepted literature on these treatments, and this often clouds the image we have of them. Note the word "accepted." Some of these treatments will generate a mountain of hits when you enter their names in your search engine.

Their effectiveness has been questioned and accusations of possible abuse have been made. The abuse is generally related to "taking advantage" of critically ill patients with unapproved or unproven treatments. The good news is, most doctors offering chelation-type options are good, caring folk who have produced impressive results with *some* patients.

I want to take a moment to cover chelation therapy in more detail, partly because it is one of the alternative treatments that are often attacked and partly because I believe it was a tremendous help to me, based not only on how I feel but on a review of the regular test results generated while I was having it.

Chelation therapy is a process involving the use of chelating agents to remove heavy metals from the body. For the most common forms of heavy metal intoxication, those involving lead, arsenic or mercury, the standard of care in the US dictates the use of DMSA. This, in addition to other chelating agents such as DMPS and alpha lipoic acid (ALA), are used in conventional and alternative medicine.[17]

EDTA and DMPS are often used in addition to DMSA. Vitamins, minerals, and other ingredients are typically added to the chelation intravenous bag (often a saline base). Given that chelation is the standard of care for some metal toxicity, I find it odd that some doctors, particularly heart doctors, seem to be so upset about its off-label use. I realize the clinical evidence is sparse (see the LDN case study in chapter nine, especially the part on money) and what does exist is questioned regularly. But the anecdotal evidence appears strong.

I have personally spoken to a couple of dozen patients who have used chelation for heart and circulation issues (including those associated with diabetes) and most of them believe it was the only thing that worked. Many felt it saved their lives. Some stated they had been sent home to put their affairs in order by more mainstream doctors. Some had been deemed poor candidates for bypass surgery or stints, while others had already had those operations but were still in real trouble. The effect on heart and circulation seems to be a welcome "side effect" of chelation. Unexpected and positive side effects are often the way new applications for treatments are found.

Since my use of chelation was targeting mercury toxicity, I can't speak personally about its effectiveness on anything else. What I can urge you to do is fire up your search engine and do some serious

---

17   http://en.wikipedia.org/wiki/Chelation_therapy

reading on it. Be advised there really is a ton of information and a lot of opinions out there. Be sure to try reading a balanced sampling, and definitely have a look at as many patient testimonials (good and bad) as you can find. Beware of fear-mongering because this issue involves tremendously high stakes not only health-wise but dollar-wise.

Many of these box docs were unhappy using allopathic tools alone. They are typically big on testing. And, as doctors, they often have more access to testing than alternative practitioners. They are also typically concerned with how your environment and diet have affected your health.

The fact they can tailor treatments to include some of this specialty stuff along with testing and prescription medication may really increase your options. It certainly increased mine and I'm grateful for that. Box docs are also more versatile in their diagnostic and treatment options because they are able to involve a specialist when needed. When you receive a scary diagnosis, options are what you need, and these are ones you should know about and understand.

Almost by definition, out-of-the-box docs are more open-minded than many more mainstream doctors. They have to be because they generally have allowed their experience to challenge some of what they were taught, and therefore use treatments not taught in medical school.

They often combine a mix of old-time remedies and practices with modern medicine. They generally top this off with a touch of what are often considered gray-area or specialty techniques, and finish with a healthy dose of common sense. Surprisingly, "gray area" includes the investigation of either deficiencies in, or overloads on, your body.

These doctors don't just address symptoms but look for causes or triggers as well. Because they're treating the body as a whole rather than always breaking it down into specialized regions or pieces, part of their research includes things considered not part of the normal evaluation or treatment process. They typically look at deficiencies and overload — vitamins, minerals, heavy metals, and chemicals being good examples. Often addressing these issues requires a process rather than a pill. This process is often a slow one that requires monitoring, and that means more tests. For me, the more tests (information) the better. Tests are good.

Occasionally patients do see fast and sometimes remarkable results from relatively simple treatments. Here's an interesting example. I sat next to an older gentleman named Frank several times while we were both receiving chelation. Since the process takes several hours, we had lots of time to talk. Frank was in his mid-80s. He told me his feet started turning black when he was in his mid-50s, apparently the result of poor circulation. (Frank was a very heavy smoker as well.) He was the president of a company and had the means to get the best medical advice available. After seeing several specialists, he was told his feet would become gangrenous and would eventually kill him if he didn't have them amputated.

So Frank began the process and surgery was scheduled. He was also given a book about chelation by a friend. Based on his reading, he scheduled an appointment with the doctor we currently were both using. The box doc felt very confident he could address the issue without removing Frank's feet. After seven treatments his feet started to look more normal. He went back to the surgeons, who declared it to be a miracle. Frank told them about the chelation but they felt the treatment had nothing to do with it.

Frank continued the treatment and then went on a long-term maintenance program, going several times a year. He continued to play golf, walking 18 holes three times a week into his late 70s, and still plays 9 holes three times a week although he now uses a golf cart. As far as I know, Frank still has his feet and is still playing golf. It's important to mention that in addition to quitting smoking he also changed his diet to a very healthy one high in fruits, vegetables, and nuts.

Box docs are trying to help you get better by giving your body (and sometimes your mind and spirit — no eye rolling, please) the right tools or by removing obstacles in order to allow your body to work the way it was designed to do.

They often accomplish this by doing more and *different* tests, using additional techniques, and asking questions probing areas such as your emotions, life choices, and attitudes. This makes sense. It's becoming more and more obvious that our health and wellness are affected by what we say, think, and believe. This has to do with what is called the mind-body connection.

MY OWN OUT-OF-THE-BOX EXPERIENCE

When I first went to a box doc, I had already done a fair bit of research and had serious questions, not only about my diagnosis but also about why nutrition and digestion weren't part of the search to confirm and treat my condition. I was able to use part of the information I had found to devise a comprehensive approach to getting better. In any case, I felt if this approach didn't make me better, it could at least make me feel better.

I had read about several dietary regimens and supplements that had shown favorable results with MS patients in many places, including the UK, but they were considered irrelevant here. These included the so-called Swank Diet and another called the Best Bet Diet. Supplements included B_{12}, turmeric (curcumin), calcium, and others.

They were considered irrelevant not only by the neurologists I had seen but by the many MS societies (yes, there are lots of them) in North America. I had come across similar information about diet and lifestyle impacting some cancers and heart issues. I'm not talking about some of the basic dietary theories regarding low fat and the like, but about specific, targeted food and nutrition issues that consider certain foods as part of your treatment.

An example is juicing fresh fruits and vegetables.

I had been searching for a doctor open-minded enough to at least humor me by helping me get answers to my many questions. I had a list of tests considered potentially relevant to confirming my diagnosis by eliminating other illnesses. These included tests for B_{12} deficiency, Lyme disease, Hughes syndrome, and mercury toxicity, to name a few.

I just kept asking everyone (doctors, friends, and acquaintances) if they knew of a doctor who was open to working with patients. I was willing to travel and knew it could end up costing me a lot, but nothing seemed more important than knowing, the best I could, what was happening to me.

All this research began to help me understand the type of doctor I was really looking for. After a few months, I ended up getting a recommendation to a doctor. Amazingly, at the same time, I found some commentary on the Internet recommending the very same doctor.

Although Dr. Paul Cutler seemed to prefer saying he practiced alternative medicine, he is an M.D. (in both the U.S. and Canada). I later realized his strong faith in chelation therapy may have put him slightly beyond the definition of integrative medicine, although he was concerned with nutrition and lifestyle as well.

Quite frankly, I didn't care what he called himself. I was determined to at least investigate any and all reasonable possibilities, and his approach seemed reasonable to me. Incredibly, Dr. Cutler had just opened a satellite office in the very town where I live. We'll have to put off any conversations about coincidence for another book.

Not only was this new box doc willing to order most of the tests I requested, but he also generated a list of his own. He took notes during my visits, using carbon paper to make a copy for me.

That alone sold me on the guy.

Even before I underwent any treatment, it was obvious to me he was thinking and practicing out of the box. I was already feeling a bit better. I dubbed him an out-of-the-box doc after my second visit. I may be the originator of this snappy phrase (just for the record).

Word of mouth is very important when looking for doctors. You want to know that they know their stuff and that they seem interested and involved with each and every patient. It may take some asking, but don't be surprised if you find a box doc close to home. Your family doctor may know of one. You'll probably need to ask rather than expecting a name to be offered, because many doctors have some issues with box docs or at least with some of the treatments they use. But when it comes to a scary diagnosis, your family doctor may be more willing to recommend someone who is less conventional, particularly if they've heard that the out-of-the-box doc has had some results with tough cases or cases similar to yours.

In addition, you can search the Internet for them.

Use your search engine and search words like "M.D." and "integrated," "alternative," "natural," "holistic," or "chelation." Add the name of your town or the closest city to narrow down the number of hits you get. It may help to add your state or province, or even your country.

Here's the standard warning.

There are good box docs and bad ones. Unfortunately the behavior of the bad ones, or bad results associated with one of their treatments, often become representative of these maverick doctors as a group. All medicine has both good and bad results. Remember Vioxx? Be sure to do your homework yourself and formulate your own opinions of good and bad.

Most doctors may be smart, but very few are the complete package. The package you're looking for includes a combination of book learning, experience, people skills, and the ability and willingness to focus on the patient.

You want someone who is aware of new developments but is not afraid to use a simple and often old-time remedy if it is appropriate and effective. You want someone who will be interested in your case. You may have to help the doctor get interested. I guarantee that if you keep records and bring them with you, do your research, and ask questions, they will become interested; if not, you need to switch doctors.

Make sure you talk to your doctor's or prospective doctor's current patients. Most box docs will be open to your chatting with some of their patients because they are sensitive to the fact that you may not be comfortable or familiar with some of what they do. They are also aware that sometimes their peers (other local doctors) may say suggestive or downright slanderous stuff about them, more often based on supposition or lack of information than on fact.

These conversations can happen in the waiting room, as it is very rare to find a doctor of any flavor who doesn't make you and others wait. Sometimes there are large rooms in which patients receive treatments that take time, like intravenous chelation. You will want to talk to a cross-section of patients, established and new, young and mature.

Try to find patients with issues similar to yours and ask about treatments, results, how they feel, what they don't like, and whether they would recommend the doctor to a loved one. Sorry, once again I am asking you to do some work. But when you're dealing with a health issue, it is downright dangerous to allow yourself to be led by *anyone*.

Take the lead and take control of making the important decisions based on being an informed "consumer."

A final note before moving on is another caution.

You certainly need to be cautious about any treatment or medication — how it might interact with other stuff you're doing, or its impact on your health and welfare in general. Do your homework and make an educated decision.

When you begin to look beyond mainstream medicine, you'll find some very pointed and direct attacks against some doctors, practitioners, and treatments. It is important to read them, but remember that just because someone wrote it doesn't make it true, especially in every case or all the time.

I have read several scathing commentaries on some of the treatments I have studied and doctors I have read about. Sometimes testing and verification will prove these criticisms to be true, sometimes quite the opposite.

Be sure to make the extra effort to convince yourself whether a criticism is fair and accurate or the work of some self-serving individual or group. Remember, the Internet is anonymous and it can be difficult to confirm who is who and whether people are what they say they are. It's also hard to know who, if anyone, is paying them (directly or indirectly) to say what they're saying, and why.

When you're ill there are more bad folks out there looking to take advantage of you than you'd like to believe. Some mean well but may have bad or incomplete information. Some seem to have their own hidden agendas. Some are just greedy and therefore despicable. Don't get discouraged by this — just get that much more focused on reaching the point where you, and not they, are making your decisions.

Don't give anyone the power to make decisions for you, whether by choice or inaction, unless it is a loved one making the same kind of effort and informed decision that you would make for yourself if you could.

INTEGRATIVE MEDICINE

There is an interesting and growing phenomenon called integrative medicine, whereby some practitioners of mainstream medicine have begun to incorporate less mainstream treatments into their practices. They may do this by themselves, but typically they form or become part of a practice or clinic that has a blend of allopathic and alternative doctors and practitioners. Some are box docs and some aren't.

The goal of integrative medicine is to address the whole body as opposed to individual issues. In this way these doctors expect to see the body use its own restorative powers to help the patient either feel better or get better. Here, from his website, is Dr. Andrew Weil's take on this phenomenon.

What is Integrative Medicine?

Integrative medicine is healing-oriented medicine that takes account of the whole person (body, mind, and spirit), including all aspects of lifestyle. It emphasizes the therapeutic relationship and makes use of all appropriate therapies, both conventional and alternative.

The principles of integrative medicine:

- A partnership between patient and practitioner in the healing process
- Appropriate use of conventional and alternative methods to facilitate the body's innate healing response
- Consideration of all factors that influence health, wellness and disease, including mind, spirit and community as well as body
- A philosophy that neither rejects conventional medicine nor accepts alternative therapies uncritically
- Recognition that good medicine should be based in good science, be inquiry driven, and be open to new paradigms
- Use of natural, effective, less-invasive interventions whenever possible
- Use of the broader concepts of promotion of health and the prevention of illness as well as the treatment of disease
- Training of practitioners to be models of health and healing, committed to the process of self-exploration and self-development[18]

Taking advantage of an integrated approach may mean more work, and it may not provide the easiest short-term answers (like "take this pill and hope for the best"), but it may result in a far better long-term prognosis. It may also limit some of the running around from office to office, given the nature of this team approach.

---

18   http://www.drweil.com/

OSTEOPATHY

Another sort of mixed doctor is a doctor of osteopathy. I believe most doctors actually practiced a form of osteopathy before we formally had drugs.

The definition and scope of this type of practice seem to vary. In the United States these doctors are also medical doctors and are called doctors of osteopathy (D.O.). In Canada, the United Kingdom, Australia, and New Zealand osteopaths are generally part of a separate practice and are not necessarily medical doctors.

In any case, what they do is practice a fascinating whole-body or "holistic" approach to illness. Consider this definition: "Osteopathic medicine is a system of health care based on the premise that disease is the result of the relationship between anatomical structure and physiological function."[19]

They may or may not like to use the term "integrative medicine" to describe what they do in their individual practices. They use physical manipulation as part of their toolkit. Some of the manipulations are different from the kind chiropractors use, but it seems to me chiropractors are essentially a subset of osteopathy.

Some illnesses seem to respond particularly well to this approach and it's worth doing some reading on it with respect to your condition. In the u.s., you get the benefit of conventional medical strategies coupled with osteopathic tools and philosophies.

I have been seeing an osteopath of late and find his work fascinating and helpful. I have high hopes that my numb side will continue to improve. I can't wait to see if my eye benefits as well.

---

19 www.footnotesforhealth.com/definitions.html

The osteopath I am seeing, Dr. Glenn Sprague, has an outstanding reputation and was recommended to me by a friend who is one of his patients. This friend suffered for years and was "cured" after an adjustment apparently repositioned a joint that was out of place. Many doctors prior to this had failed to find or fix this particular problem. Since he was a carpet layer and was often using his knee and hip to stretch carpets to fit properly, getting this problem resolved not only meant no more pain, but also that he could happily continue his work.

ALTERNATIVE MEDICINE

Chiropractic

I know many chiropractors (chiros) are not going to be happy that I have sort of grouped them under alternative medicine, but I believe they will be pleased with what I have to say (so no letters, emails, phone calls, or faxes, please).

I, for one, no longer consider most chiropractors practitioners of alternative medicine.

Some folks love chiros and some don't. Some chiros are good at what they do and some simply aren't. I believe, based on personal experience, certain conditions are best treated through some kind of manipulation, by either a chiropractor or an osteopath. Some chiros provide a holistic approach. Others focus only on adjustments.

I do have to wonder if there may be too many chiropractors in some areas these days. Offices seem to open up on almost every corner. Perhaps this is only true in the places I've lived, but I don't think so. I'm guessing that the number of chiropractors in a given area often results in some of them having to branch out into things like supplements, laser treatments, and weight loss.

It is not up to me to say whether this diversification is good or bad. As a patient who has seen five or six different ones over the years, I know what's important is the quantity and quality of the chiropractic service I receive. Personal care comes first. The add-ons may not even be relevant.

There's more than one kind of chiropractic manipulation technique. Different chiros use different techniques. Some use tables that move, and some mainly use a tool called an activator. Most use a mix of several tools and techniques.

I personally prefer "soft" and often subtle adjustments, or the use of an activator, as opposed to more active or aggressive maneuvers or tables that move.

Sometimes a symptom may not be directly related to your condition but may become an issue because you're sitting more than you used to, or spending more time on your computer searching the Internet for options (sorry, but it's worth it). Chiropractors are often a viable option for helping you feel a bit better. Because adjustments are physical in nature, you may need to see one regularly to keep things properly aligned in your body. I believe this is much better than taking a drug, any drug, long-term.

Take a moment to type in the name of your condition or illness and the word "chiropractor" into your Internet search engine and see what pops up. As a result of doing this myself, I now have my chiropractor check certain things for my MS diagnosis and can typically tell when a slight adjustment is needed.

In my case, I believe these adjustments help.

My experience provides an additional example of a chiropractor addressing problems that we may not normally associate with adjustments. My wife, Deborah, was experiencing bouts of vertigo (extreme dizziness). Our family doctor said he could prescribe something, but that results were rarely satisfactory. He noted that in extreme cases there were some surgical approaches that might help, but they didn't sound good to her.

He suggested she try to just live with it and hope it would go away.

When I mentioned the situation to my chiropractor, he said to have her come in immediately. He put a rubber glove on and adjusted something in her mouth. She says she was 70% better almost immediately. A couple of days later she had a second glove-in-mouth adjustment and was almost 100% better.

I asked Dr. Brian Smuk to comment on this adjustment. Here's what he had to say:

> Among the many causes of vertigo — viral, vestibular, vestibular-cochlear, benign-positional, and many others — the one I see most is TMJ-related. More specifically, the vertigo is related to aberrant tension on either side of the jaw. When resting tension in the jaw muscles is too high, especially when the tension is one-sided, there is compression or compaction against the temperomandibular joint. When that pressure is increased, you can end up with episodic vertigo. This is the same principle at work, though to a larger, more dramatic extent, when a knockout punch is delivered in boxing. Hitting the jaw and compacting the joint causes severe loss of equilibrium, even to the point of loss of consciousness. In the episodic type of vertigo, the therapeutic goal is to reduce resting tension of the jaw muscles to reduce the compaction on the TMJ. By first muscle testing to determine which muscles are involved, we can direct treatment to the correct area. Several muscles are involved in closing the jaw. In some cases,

the best access to physically manipulating the correct muscle is to go into the mouth rather than making an adjustment on the outer, more superficial jaw muscles.

The problem with vertigo stayed away for some time and now she occasionally goes in for readjustment as needed. No drugs. No surgery. No living with it and hoping it goes away.

It's worth noting there was also no referral from our doctor, or even a hint there was such a simple and effective option. I'm guessing he didn't know such an "adjustment" existed.

Here's another example involving my wife — another problem I would never have thought a chiropractor could address. I assumed some kind of drug had to be the solution.

My wife had a bad flu. In addition to her other symptoms, she was experiencing severe diarrhea. Our chiro pressed deep into my wife's right side and adjusted her ileocecal valve, and that stopped her diarrhea.

Again, here's what Dr. Brian has to say:

The digestive system consists of three main areas: stomach, small intestine, and large intestine. The small intestine can be further divided into three divisions: the duodenum, jejunum, and ileum. Where the ileum meets the large intestine (the first part of it is called the cecum), there is a valve, a door that opens and closes to allow waste to move into the large intestine when necessary. This is called the ileocecal valve (icv). Many things — nutritional irritants, toxins, certain nerve conditions, and many others — can cause this doorway to misfunction. This results in three main types of problems.

Problem one is that substances move too quickly through the small intestine and run right into the large. When this happens, diarrhea usually results and sufferers are not able to go too far from the bathroom immediately after eating. Things are moving much too quickly. The biggest problem with this is malabsorption of nutrients from food. This will often be diagnosed as some kind of "irritable" condition or any number of medical "syndromes."

Problem two is the opposite. Substances get stuck at the ICV, waiting for it to open. But the ICV does not open when it should and there is a backlog of waste that's not getting to the large intestine. When the door does open, it only opens a small amount and for a limited time. The result is a distinct lack of normal bowel movements often described as rabbit pellets. This results in bloating, fluid retention, headaches, mental fog, and an uncomfortable full feeling. As you retain wastes there is reabsorption of them into the bloodstream causing an auto toxicity — basically a poisoning of the self with one's own wastes.

Problem three is a combination of the above problems. Sometimes the ICV is stuck open and sometimes it is stuck closed. Usually there is a specific trigger for this, such as a severe food sensitivity. A person experiencing problem three is always uncomfortable, alternating between diarrhea and constipation, never really getting to any middle ground.

Good testing and assessment are imperative with these conditions because there are many causes and many corrections. Chasing a symptom or two without looking at overall health, diet pattern, lifestyle, and signs and symptoms usually leads to many misdiagnoses. As with any condition, each case is very specific to the individual. You could see ten people with the same signs and symptoms but upon testing find ten different causes.

Once the diarrhea was stopped, she recovered quickly. Who knew?

Since some chiros are more skilled or just plain better at their profession than others, you need to shop around to find one who best suits your needs. If they require an x-ray before treating you, make sure they understand you will be taking the film with you after they've read it.

Ask for referrals from friends and family. I thought I had a good one until I started seeing Dr. Brian. The difference, in time spent with me and in his overall skill, is like night and day.

Since chiropractic practices are businesses, some chiropractors want to maximize the number of patients they see in a day. Their goal is to "rack 'em and crack 'em."

But as my wife and I discovered, there are some who are more focused on individual results, and they will often spend the extra time and make the extra effort to become an important part of your long-term health and wellness team. This is where the sheer number of chiropractors can be of benefit to you. The best advice I can give you is to try different ones until you find the right one for you.

It's yet again more work, but it can really be worth the effort.

Colonics
Now let's get to the bottom of things. (I really couldn't resist — forgive me.)

Colonics is another alternative therapy I've tried. I've already mentioned it briefly, but it deserves a closer look.

I've had a couple of colonic treatments and can say I am certainly a lot less shy. Having a tube up your butt will do that for you. I am becoming a real believer in this treatment. I read several books on elimination and recommend *Tissue Cleansing Through Bowel Management* by Dr. Bernard Jensen. You can find some of his work on the Internet.

I'm betting that most of you who do read it and have a look at some of the pictures will be highly motivated to clean out, and fast.

Do a quick Internet search for "enemas" and "colonics," adding "who" and "why," and start reading. There are lots of folks doing this stuff, but it's obviously something typically kept somewhat private. You can add the name of your condition or diagnosis to the search to find information more relevant to you.

Talking about bowel movements is not my idea of a good time, but it may be extremely important for regaining good health as well as maintaining it.

ENERGY, FREQUENCY, AND VIBRATIONAL MEDICINE

I'm an engineer. When I first heard the terms "vibrational medicine," "frequency medicine," and "energy medicine," I thought, "Gimme a break."

Then I started reading some books on these topics. Most were about physics and were typically written by Ph.D.s or M.D.s (one I read was written by someone with both degrees). I found there were practical applications of these things and some of them were mainstream. Here's a definition:

Energy medicine is a domain in Complementary Alternative Medicine that deals with energy fields of two types:

1. Veritable, which can be measured
2. Putative, which have yet to be measured

   The veritable energies employ mechanical vibrations (such as sound) and electromagnetic forces, including visible light, magnetism, monochromatic radiation (such as laser beams), and rays from other parts of the electromagnetic spectrum. They involve the use of specific, measurable wavelengths and frequencies to treat patients.

In contrast, putative energy fields (also called biofields) have defied measurement to date by reproducible methods. Therapies involving putative energy fields are based on the concept that human beings are infused with a subtle form of energy. This vital energy or life force is known under different names in different cultures, such as qi in traditional Chinese medicine (TCM), ki in the Japanese Kampo system, doshas in Ayurvedic medicine, and elsewhere as prana, etheric energy, fohat, orgone, odic force, mana, and homeopathic resonance. Vital energy is believed to flow throughout the material human body, but it has not been unequivocally measured by means of conventional instrumentation. Nonetheless, therapists claim that they can work with this subtle energy, see it with their own eyes, and use it to effect changes in the physical body and influence health.

Practitioners of energy medicine believe that illness results from disturbances of these subtle energies (the biofield). For example, more than 2,000 years ago, Asian practitioners postulated that the flow and balance of life energies are necessary for maintaining health and described tools to restore them. Herbal medicine, acupuncture, acupressure, moxibustion, and cupping, for example, are all believed to act by correcting imbalances in the internal biofield, such as by restoring the flow of qi through meridians to reinstate health. Some therapists are believed to emit or transmit the vital energy (external qi) to a recipient to restore health.[20]

Here's a brief and certainly incomplete list of things often included under the Energy label.

---

20 http://www.wikihealth.com/Energy_medicine

- Veritable Energy Medicine
- Magnetic Therapy
- Millimeter Wave Therapy
- Sound Energy Therapy
- Light Therapy
- Energy Medicine Involving Putative Energy Fields
- Acupuncture
- Qi Gong
- Whole Medical Systems and Energy Medicine
- Homeopathy
- Therapeutic Touch and Related Practices
- Distant Healing[21]

To get a bit more specific about Veritable Energy, here's a nice summary:

> There are many well-established uses for the application of measurable energy fields to diagnose or treat diseases: electromagnetic fields in magnetic resonance imaging, cardiac pacemakers, radiation therapy, ultraviolet light for psoriasis, laser keratoplasty, and more. There are many other claimed uses as well. The ability to deliver quantifiable amounts of energies across the electromagnetic spectrum is an advantage to studies of their mechanisms and clinical effects. For example, both static and pulsating electromagnetic therapies have been employed.[22]

I have and use an electro-magnetic pulser. I bought it after reading comments from several MSers. It's used to address pain and inflammation. Em-Probe claims it can be used to address (among other things listed on their website):

---

21 http://www.wikihealth.com/Energy_medicine
22 http://www.wikihealth.com/Energy_medicine#Veritable_Energy_Medicine

Arthritis	Pain relief	Back pain
Migraine	Neck pain	Neuritis
Sciatica	Sports injury	Whiplash

The website indicates that "EMpulse circuit is FDA certified for relief of joint and muscle pain."[23]

This technology has also been studied by NASA and is in use around the world.

All of a sudden something that sounded far-fetched seemed to make perfect sense based on the "science" behind it. It also became clear I had some preconceived notions about what this stuff was that was proving incomplete and incorrect. Remember, make sure you know what the words you're reading really mean.

Before moving on I'd also like to mention TENS units. Here's a definition:

> Transcutaneous Electrical Nerve Stimulator, more commonly referred to as a TENS unit and pronounced *tens*, is an electronic device that produces electrical signals used to stimulate nerves through unbroken skin. The name was coined by Dr. Charles Burton. The unit is usually connected to the skin using two or more electrodes. A typical battery-operated TENS unit consists of a pulse generator, small transformer, frequency and intensity controls, and a number of electrodes.[24]

These units are mainly used for pain relief but also to stimulate nerves. When my arm went sort of numb and weak and the pinkie on my left hand stopped working, I had a number of treatments, including TENS sessions and acupuncture. I have to believe both of

---

23 http://www.em-probe.com/
24 http://en.wikipedia.org/wiki/Transcutaneous_Electrical_Nerve_Stimulator

those things did something because over time my arm and finger have almost returned to normal. Both are a bit weaker than I'd like, but I'm right-handed, so perhaps they're just about where they should be. I should note that some TENS units warn against using it on numb areas. It is best to read the directions (yes, I usually do) and ask when in doubt.

Here's my now standard warning: Before deciding to try anything I talk about in this book, you need to do your homework and decide, based on the best information you can find, whether or not it is right for you.

My sense is that these kinds of medicine and the technologies and practices associated with them are in their infancy even though many of the concepts are quite old and some are in regular use outside North America. And obviously some are mainstream already. Stay tuned and keep an eye on advances in Energy Medicine.

OTHER ALTERNATIVE PRACTICES

Let's step a little further out onto the fringe of conventional and alternative medicines.

Are some of the things lumped together as alternative medicine, or perhaps some of the folks who practice it, questionable? Yes.

But so are some of the mainstream treatments that come in and out of favor and so are some of the doctors who practice medicine in general.

Some things I ended up trying just made no sense but seemed to work. For example, I had a lot of applied kinesiology done on me. In its simplest form it is often referred to as "muscle testing." It wasn't so much a treatment as it was testing. By physically manipulating different muscles, the doctor seemed to be able to identify areas of my body that needed attention. I could be blind-tested against unmarked samples, and time after time the doctor could pick the same "bad" ones. It seemed it couldn't possibly work and give consistent results, yet time after time it did.

Obviously, just as with my preconceived notion that doctors knew it all and could fix me, I was once again very wrong about at least some of these alternative practices. My notions were yet again proving to be the fairy tales.

By now at least I knew better. It was time to stop believing something was so just because I had always believed it to be or because someone flippantly said so, and start asking the tough questions and paying attention to the answers. And I mean paying attention to the answers whether I liked them or not.

The following list of alternative practices, though long, is woefully incomplete. There are so many and some are so specific and exotic that they go beyond the scope of this book. But this doesn't mean that an alternative therapy not listed here should go unchecked by you.

Acupuncture	Jin Shin Do
Applied Kinesiology	Massage Therapy
Aromatherapy	Meditation
Auricular Medicine	Naturopath
Chiropractor	NLP
Colon Therapy (Colonics)	Nutritionist
Craniopathy	Prayer
Darkfield Microscopy	Pulsed Electromagnetic
Dentists (Biological)	Fields (PEMF)
Ear Coning	Orthotics
Energy Healing	Qi Gung
European Biological Medicine	Reflexology

Exercise	Reiki
Feng Shui	Tai Chi
Homeopathy	Total Body Modification
Iridology	(TBM)
	Yoga

Some of these are really quite interesting. For example, I know a man named Alexander who practices Jin Shin Do. It's sort of like acupuncture but uses pressure instead of needles. Some of his treatments have had noticeable results. Some I thought of as "exercise" but apparently they are considered by some as therapies as well.

Then there's craniopathy, which is a subtle manipulation of the bones in your head. Yes, there are 22 bones in your head. (That was news to me.) This manipulation is often done by some chiropractors or osteopaths. Again, I've had it done on occasion with sometimes noticeable effects. One time my sinuses drained and an odd feeling of relaxation seemed to permeate through me. My breath seemed to come easier and be more rhythmic. Other times it just seemed like something was put back into sync. In both cases the feeling was a bit weird but certainly welcome.

I'd also like to mention biofeedback and electro-dermal and similar devices. I have had some experience with several of them. They typically include an analysis mode listing what may be wrong with you and a treatment mode addressing the problem areas. They often use straps or probes to monitor some of your body's reaction to stimuli. They certainly seem to belong here and are often considered an energy treatment. I had a particularly bizarre experience with one of them, but since it wasn't medical, let's leave that for another time.

In your search engine, enter the words "alternative medicine" plus the name of your town or city along with any additional key words to help narrow your search. My local phone book was of little help.

Go to a health food store or the like in your area. Such places often have business cards of local practitioners. Any of a variety of specialized newspapers (typically free) or magazines may advertise loads of local choices.

It's certainly true that some alternative stuff, especially the real fringe practices, can get pretty airy-fairy and far-fetched. Some of it is. Occasionally some of it works.

I have come to learn that just because something seems far-fetched on the surface doesn't mean there may not be something sensible about it on some level, and it certainly doesn't mean it might not help you feel or even get better. No doubt some of these practices and treatments will make perfect sense and be in mainstream use in the future as our ability to understand and use them grows. When it comes to a scary diagnosis, it's best to leave no stone unturned.

NINE

A CASE STUDY: THE LDN STORY

I'm a great believer in luck, and I find the
harder I work the more I have of it.
— THOMAS JEFFERSON

SHORTLY AFTER BEGINNING my ongoing scouring of the Internet
for information to help confirm or eliminate various potential
diagnoses, I began staying up till all hours of the night lurking in
user groups populated by other MSers. They talked about diagnoses,
symptoms, doctors, treatments, drugs, and all manner of things
related to understanding what we all had and what to do about it. I
started making a list of things to research further. Things to verify
the best I could.

Sure, there was some far-fetched stuff and some companies
making amazing claims. I filed these away for future review. But
some MSers used diets, including supplements. Some used alternative
treatments, including massage, reflexology, chiropractic adjustment,
acupuncture, and other things.

One topic that kept coming up was the off-label use of a drug called Naltrexone.

I wasn't reading about it on a drug company's website or in the company's marketing material. I was reading commentary from people using it. It's referred to as Low Dose Naltrexone (LDN) when used for MS and a host of other autoimmune-related diseases. It was even being used with some reported success on some cancers and AIDS.

Originally LDN was FDA-approved in doses of 50 mg, but folks with a variety of autoimmune diseases were taking it in very low doses ranging from 1 mg to 6 mg. Most were taking it nightly at 4.5 mg. The astounding thing is that no one I had seen — not any of the many doctors, not the MS clinic — ever mentioned this drug. Yet many if not most MS patients using it were reporting significant if not fantastic results.

Patients praised LDN not only when comparing it with the "approved" MS medication, but in general. And it cost less than $30 a month, more than 30 times cheaper than the cheapest of the CRAB drugs. And it was a pill, not an injection.

Was I dreaming? Was I hallucinating? Was I just plain confused?

Not only did LDN really exist, but most people with RRMS (relapsing and remitting multiple sclerosis) seemed to believe that the drug had stopped the progression of the disease.

No progression! Not a cure, but almost the Holy Grail.

Most MSers are RRMS, which means they have "attacks" and get better, but not all the way better. This means they degrade over time. If you can slow down or stop the attacks, you may still have some past damage, but you aren't getting worse, or at least you slow your degeneration down. Some MSers are progressive, which means they are sort of under attack all the time. They are tougher to treat, but even some of them reported doing better on LDN than on anything else they had tried.

Many of the folks taking LDN had injected some or all of the CRAB drugs, along with trying all kinds of other things I didn't know about.

Why hadn't I been told about any of this other stuff?

Well, we are back to clinical trials versus anecdotal evidence. The anecdotal evidence in favor of LDN consisted of a rapidly growing group of patients reporting excellent results from taking an approved drug that wasn't approved for what they were taking it for.

The more I read about LDN, the more surrealistic the situation seemed. Not only was it an approved drug with a long history, but the potential side effects were minimal, especially at low doses. Dr. Bernard Bihari, a Harvard-educated doctor in New York, had been prescribing it for years, and not only for MS but for all kinds of things included on the following chart (the list may have grown by the time you read this):

Breast cancer	ALS (Lou Gehrig's disease)
Carcinoid	Alzheimer's disease
Colon and rectal cancer	Behcet's disease
Glioblastoma	Celiac disease
Liver cancer	Chronic Fatigue Syndrome
Lung cancer (non-small cell)	Crohn's disease
Lymphocytic leukemia	Emphysema (COPD)
Lymphoma (Hodgkin's and non-Hodgkin's)	Fibromyalgia
	HIV/AIDS
Malignant melanoma	Irritable bowel syndrome (IBS)
Multiple myeloma	Multiple sclerosis (MS)
Neuroblastoma	Parkinson's disease

Ovarian cancer	Pemphigoid
Pancreatic cancer	Primary Lateral Sclerosis (PLS)
Prostate cancer (untreated)	Psoriasis
Renal cell carcinoma	Rheumatoid arthritis
Throat cancer	Sarcoidosis
Uterine cancer	Systemic lupus (SLE)
Ulcerative colitis	Wegener's granulomatosis[25]

Now, I may consider myself plain vanilla, but that doesn't mean I'm an easy mark, nor does it mean I'm completely lacking in common sense. There were several big questions to ask and I started asking them.

TOO GOOD TO BE TRUE? BUT WHY?

I had by now joined user groups focused on LDN and had read basically everything associated with those groups, as well as scouring the LDN home page. (You can find the page by typing "LDN" into most search engines; it is often first in the list of hits. The address is http://www.lowdosenaltrexone.org/.)

It seemed LDN was useful for a lot of stuff. How could that be? Was it some kind of miracle cure-all?

I talked earlier about what I have come to believe is fundamental to illness. I believe many if not most illnesses are related in the sense that the patient doesn't become symptomatic until their "teapot" is full or, in more technical terms, until their immune system is stretched to the breaking point. Once that happens, the "triggers" (virus, bacteria, fungus, or parasite), your genetic predispositions (weak spots), and your overall health and wellness dictate what you end up getting diagnosed with.

---

25 Low Dose Naltrexone website: www.lowdosenaltrexone.org

Take a good look at the list of illnesses that LDN may be helpful in treating. Common sense would dictate, if you agree with my simplified view of illness, that it was at least reasonable that LDN would be helpful for some if not all conditions on this fairly diverse list.

Think about how many things some people take medications for. Aspirin or other over-the-counter drugs often seem to be touted as cure-alls. If many of the illnesses listed on the LDN site had inflammation- or immune-related issues associated with them, which they do, then it seemed very possible that LDN could be effective even across this seemingly diverse list.

The following is taken from the LDN home page and explains how LDN is thought to work.

How does LDN work?

LDN boosts the immune system, activating the body's own natural defenses.

Up to the present time, the question of "What controls the immune system?" has not been present in the curricula of medical colleges and the issue has not formed a part of the received wisdom of practicing physicians. Nonetheless, a body of research over the past two decades has pointed repeatedly to one's own endorphin secretions (our internal opioids) as playing the central role in the beneficial orchestration of the immune system, and recognition of the facts is growing.

Witness these statements from a recent review article of medical progress in the November 13, 2003 issue of the prestigious *New England Journal of Medicine*: "Opioid-Induced Immune Modulation: ... Preclinical evidence indicates overwhelmingly that opioids alter the development, differentiation, and function of immune cells, and that both innate and adaptive systems are affected. Bone marrow progenitor cells, macro-phages, natural killer cells, immature thymocytes and T cells, and B cells are all involved. The relatively recent identification of opioid-related receptors on immune cells makes it even more likely that opioids have direct effects on the immune system."

The brief blockade of opioid receptors between 2 a.m. and 4 a.m. that is caused by taking LDN at bedtime each night is believed to produce a prolonged up-regulation of vital elements of the immune system by causing an increase in endorphin and enkephalin production. Normal volunteers who have taken LDN in this fashion have been found to have much higher levels of beta-endorphins circulating in their blood in the following days. Animal research by I. Zagon, Ph.D., and his colleagues has shown a marked increase in metenkephalin levels as well.

Bihari says that his patients with HIV/AIDS who regularly took LDN before the availability of HAART were generally spared any deterioration of their important helper T cells (CD4+).

In human cancer, research by Zagon over many years has demonstrated inhibition of a number of different human tumors in laboratory studies by using endorphins and low dose naltrexone. It is suggested that the increased endorphin and enkephalin levels, induced by LDN, work directly on the tumors' opioid receptors — and, perhaps, induce cancer cell death (apoptosis). In addition, it is believed that they act to increase natural killer cells and other healthy immune defenses against cancer.

In general, in people with diseases that are partially or largely triggered by a deficiency of endorphins (including cancer and autoimmune diseases), or are accelerated by a deficiency of endorphins (such as HIV/AIDS), restoration of the body's normal production of endorphins is the major therapeutic action of LDN.[26]

Is this reasonable? Is this possible? I think so. It's at least as reasonable as anything I've read about my other options.

The next big question was why so few doctors seemed to know about LDN or so few were willing to prescribe it once they did. My first neurologist, after a bit of probing by me, owned up to the fact he had heard about it but wouldn't touch it because it wasn't approved for MS. He is the same guy who didn't want to be labeled a "marijuana doctor." I had already thought about asking for a referral to a more aggressive, cutting-edge neurologist, preferably one associated with clinical trials, and after this I knew for sure I needed to move on.

In the meantime, I printed out a bunch of stuff about LDN and took it to my family doctor. Family doctors seem more open to writing an off-label prescription because they write so many prescriptions for such a wide variety of things. They are also more focused on what works because they generally have more of a relationship with their patients.

A specialist like a neurologist, on the other hand, tends to write much fewer prescriptions and for a much smaller number of drugs.

My doctor was intrigued and after reading the material told me he would write a prescription if need be. His logic was that it was an approved drug with a long history and few side effects. He seemed to think that while LDN in low doses might not help me, it certainly wouldn't hurt me.

---

26 www.lowdosenaltrexone.org

I thanked him and told him I planned to send copies of all my records and films to the neurologist in New York who first started using LDN for MS. I hoped he would see me and prescribe LDN for me. This made sense to my doctor because he had no experience with LDN and little with MS.

I sent copies of all my tests and films to New York and soon after a long telephone consultation with the "father" of LDN I got my first pills. I must say this telephone consultation in many ways was more complete, focused, and informative than many I had had in person.

I believe it was in April, almost three months after my left eye went fuzzy, that I started taking LDN.

I waited more than three months to see my second neurologist locally (the third if you include the one I had the phone consultation with). He was the head of the neurology department in a hospital I had never been to before. He had written a book on MS and certainly seemed more attuned to things happening beyond the good old SOC (standard of care, if you forgot). I had three looseleaf binders full of information, copies of my films, of my reports, and of the conflicting reports from the radiologists, and loads of information on LDN.

After a brief exam and some discussion about all I had learned, my new and now current neurologist immediately admitted hearing of LDN. In fact, he even knew about the doctor in New York. He also "thought" he might have a couple of patients taking LDN. Being a professional he didn't want to talk about his other patients.

But he had not written a prescription for it for anyone to date.

He asked me what I wanted to do based on all I had learned. I told him I wanted to stay on LDN and not go on a CRAB drug. To his credit, he told me that it was not SOC but he would go along with my decision and continue to see me as needed or once a year.

When I saw him a second time, for my one-year review, he told me he had at least five patients on LDN and I believe he is now at least open to prescribing it, although you may need to ask him for LDN as opposed to his offering it.

He also couldn't get over how well I was doing. I had not progressed and I had even seen some improvement in old damage.

My first neurologist had made it clear that if I rejected SOC and used LDN, he was unwilling to expose himself to the risks of potential litigation, blacklisting (real or imaginary) by his colleagues, or the extra work a non-standard patient might mean.

Don't settle for a doctor who is willing to admit to being more interested in themselves than in you.

It's a really bad sign.

ALWAYS FOLLOW THE MONEY

The next issue, in retrospect, seems a bit ridiculous.

All the approved MS drugs were very expensive. LDN was so cheap. Could something so inexpensive possibly be as good as or even better than the expensive stuff?

Of course price shouldn't have much bearing on how well LDN did or didn't work, but we live in a world where too many of us have odd notions about price. It turns out the patent protection for Naltrexone ran out long ago and the drug is available as a generic as well.

Not only that, but pricing was initially based on 50 mg pills whereas most LDN users take pills of 3 mg or 4.5 mg. In order to get the low doses, we need to fill our prescriptions at compounding pharmacies. (See the previous chapter for more on these pharmacies.)

This clinical trial thing was an issue as well. Or was it? If LDN was working, why weren't there some clinical trials going on? Most LDN users will point you to the money again. LDN is cheap and out of patent protection. Remember, clinical trials are often paid for by the drug company holding the patents, and positive trials help them sell lots of their drugs.

Is the clinical trial concept that much better than anecdotal evidence? In a perfect world, probably so, but as we discussed earlier, the world of clinical trials ain't perfect. So if the money part of doing trials didn't make sense to the people who typically pay for them, why would anyone want to do them?

Sure, the patients, the people taking LDN, wanted trials so there would be more information about LDN and so it would be readily available and offered to everyone as an option.

But who can make money, and I mean serious money, on a cheap drug that is past patent protection and available as a generic? And how much money compared with other more expensive and "younger" drugs (still patent protected)? LDN costs me about a dollar a day — peanuts compared with the prices charged for the "approved" MS drugs.

Fire up your search engines and do some reading. There's more good news here. There are some clinical trials happening and others being considered for LDN. One on LDN and Crohn's disease, a couple on MS, and others. Some are happening because universities got involved. Others are happening or are being considered because LDN users are banding together and writing, as well as raising money.

Raising money, you say? Yes, through donations and fundraising on the Internet.

WILL YOU GET LUCKY, TOO?

LDN is not a cure. Is it working for me? I believe so.

In my case I'm taking it to slow down or stop attacks. It has been almost three years since the attack that led to my diagnosis, and I believe I have not had an attack or any progression of my condition since.

In fact, I have had some improvement in old symptoms. Some improvement has been reported by some LDN users but it is considered a bonus if and when that happens. Most of us are happy just to stay stable. I'm one of the very lucky ones. My damage isn't too bad and not readily noticeable.

Because I don't know whether or when I would have had an attack, it is hard to say about any one thing, including LDN, that it's working at all. I believe it is, but only time will tell. Of course, the same thing can be said about any MS medication, including the CRAB drugs, which claim a 30% likelihood of *reducing* attacks.

In addition, I have tried countless other treatments, but LDN is the only drug I take related to MS. I did change my diet and eating habits significantly, I do take supplements, I sleep lots (when I can), and try to exercise (at least walk). All of which helps.

After reading this you may ask how I can attribute my good condition to LDN. Maybe it's the placebo effect.

I can't definitively attribute my current condition, at least not wholly, to LDN. It may be the placebo effect, but I am here to tell you I don't care. My reason for taking it wasn't to prove it works, or why it works, or how it works. My goal was and is to remain as stable and healthy as possible. Proving it works, well, that's what clinical trials are for, right?

I would love to know why things have gone so well for me, but all I really care about is that they have. I believe I'll take LDN as long as I live unless something better comes along, and I will continue to do and try things that make sense to me. I hope I'm convincing you to do the same.

TEN

A CASE STUDY: THE TROUBLE WITH DENTISTRY

Some tortures are physical and some are mental,
but the one that is both is dental.
— OGDEN NASH

WHEN I WAS first planning this book I had a feeling my comments on milk (see next chapter) would garner me the most negative comments, but now I'm thinking I was wrong. It will probably be what I say about dentistry in this chapter.

That grief will probably be only short-term, however, because these issues will be mainstream on Main Street before long. Some already are.

THE MOUTH AND HEALTH

Since digestion starts with chewing, the mouth should get honorable mention in any overview of wellness and health.

The long-term effects of what happens in the mouth with respect to major illnesses are often hotly debated. But now that the relationship between certain heart-related plaques and bacteria residing in your mouth has been repeatedly demonstrated, the door is open to taking a much better look at how your body responds to what's put into, and what lives in, your mouth. And also what your dentists have put in there through the years.

If you have an ongoing health issue of any kind, you should take a long, hard look at anything related to brushing (especially toothpastes), flossing, dental visits, related chemicals, and certainly mercury fillings, along with any other metal or "dental material" in your mouth. You also need to take a serious look at root canals.

I have come to believe that when it comes to illness, oral hygiene and dental care most certainly play a far more important role than the general public is aware. I'm not just talking about the health of our teeth and gums but about our entire body.

There's mounting evidence that many scary diagnoses can be traced in one way or another to the mouth. If you're interested in the illness-mouth connection, you'll find tons of information on the Internet and in a growing number of books.

Not so long ago, people questioning common dental practices were made to think they were foolish or even crazy. Today, in dentistry, the relationship between mouth and illness is becoming a hot topic. If you have any doubts, do a quick search of "dentistry" and "health issues." I just did and got over 19 million hits. Adding "heart" to my search knocked the number down to over seven million. Searching for "dentistry" and "multiple sclerosis" generated almost four million, and "dentistry" and "Alzheimer's" about 500,000 fewer than that.

I believe lots of additional cause-and-effect relationships involving illness, the mouth, and dentistry will be surfacing regularly from here on in as we learn more through increased communications and access to information, beginning with the Internet. We will also learn more as our understanding of the human genome increases and the tools with which we look at and evaluate the smallest of the small components of life improve.

It won't be long before some of these dental issues will be getting a lot more play on news shows, allowing us to hear (and actually believe) more about this very serious issue. I added the "and actually believe" part because my research has taught me that the best science of the day may suggest that something is likely to be a fact, but until the media embrace it, few end up hearing about it and even fewer apparently choose to believe it. All too often this includes doctors.

Till now few have chosen to tackle head-on the often subtle issues associated with overall health and dentistry. It is very difficult to prove definitively that dental-related triggers are involved in a whole host of scary diagnoses. But as more and more folks become symptomatic and ill, the taboos preventing public focus on heavy metals, root canals, fluoride treatments, some whitening programs, some of the new plastics and related solvents, and the mouth in general will be forced to give way.

MERCURY AND THE MOUTH

In the dentist's office, mercury gets mixed into an amalgam and is pressed and drilled. Being exposed to mercury in a dentist's office can happen in the air or from direct contact with your mouth — and who hasn't swallowed some of it? Then it sits in your mouth, an acidic environment, for 20 or 30 years getting pounded every time you chew. Cracks develop and pieces break off. Vapors get created and you breathe them in.

But the American Dental Association and the Canadian Dental Association know, they *know*, this highly toxic substance is safe for long-term use and exposure (just like others know that vaccinations are safe long-term).

At one time mercury fillings or amalgams were represented as absolutely safe. In many places they are still said to be. I once got a real scolding from my dentist (ex-dentist, that is) just for asking about their safety. Here is a basic definition of mercury:

mer·cu·ry (mûrky-r)
n.
1. *Symbol* **Hg** A silvery-white poisonous metallic element, liquid at room temperature and used in thermometers, barometers, vapor lamps, and batteries and in the preparation of chemical pesticides. Atomic number 80; atomic weight 200.59; melting point -38.87°C; boiling point 356.58°C; specific gravity 13.546 (at 20°C); valence 1, 2. Also called *quicksilver.*[27]

Following is a partial reproduction of information related to mercury on the Centers for Disease Control (CDC) website:

Mercury (Organic)
Clinical description

Although ingestion of organic mercury is the most typical route of organic mercury toxicity, toxicity might also result from inhalation and dermal exposures, particularly with dimethylmercury. Symptoms of toxicity are typically delayed for > 1 month after organic mercury exposure and usually involve the central nervous system. These symptoms might include paresthesias, headaches, ataxia, dysarthria, visual field constriction, blindness, and hearing impairment.[28]

---

27 http://www.thefreedictionary.com/mercury
28 http://www.bt.cdc.gov/agent/mercury/mercorgcasedef.asp

Here's some additional information on mercury poisoning from MedicineNet.com:

Definition of Mercury Poisoning

Mercury Poisoning: The metallic element mercury is poisonous to humans. Mercury poisoning can occur in both acute and chronic forms.

Acute mercury poisoning (which today is less common) is associated with ulcerations of the stomach and intestine and with toxic changes in the renal (kidney) tubules. Anuria (failure to form urine) and anemia may occur.

Chronic mercury poisoning can cause diarrhea, slowed reflexes, poor coordination, ataxia (wobbliness), tremor, impaired vision, and emotional instability.

Death and illness from mercury poisoning have long been recognized. The expression "mad as a hatter" came from the occupational hazard of hat makers in the 1800's who were poisoned by mercury salts used in the making of felt hats. Consumption of food contaminated with methyl mercury in the second half of the 20th century resulted in death or illness for thousands of people around Minimata Bay, Japan.

Minamata disease is, in fact, the name of a disorder caused by methyl mercury poisoning that was first described in the inhabitants of Minamata Bay and resulted from their eating fish contaminated with mercury industrial waste. The disease is characterized by peripheral sensory loss, tremors, dysarthria, ataxia, and both hearing and visual loss.

Even the unborn child is at risk from Minimata disease. Methyl mercury readily crosses the placenta from mother to fetus and is teratogenic, particularly to the developing brain. Children born with Minimata disease can have growth deficiency, microcephaly (an abnormally small head), severe mental retardation and be deaf and blind.

Minimata disease has not been confined to Minimata where the source of the mercury was primarily from eating fish caught in the contaminated Bay. Other sources of maternal exposure to methyl mercury have included flour made from seed grain treated with methyl mercury (which affected at least 6,500 people in Iraq) and meat from animals raised on mercury-tainted grain (in New Mexico, USA).

Mercury is discharged into the air by such sources as coal-burning power plants, incinerators, and mining. It eventually contaminates waterways where it is converted by bacteria into methylmercury. This molecule collects in the fatty tissues of fish and the animals that eat fish. Fish are the major dietary source of mercury, but it can also enter the body in other ways including diet, dental fillings, pharmaceuticals and contact with mercury metal or its compounds.

The U.S. Food and Drug Administration (FDA) as of 1999 recommends limiting consumption to 1 kilogram (2.2 pounds) of fish and shellfish a week and considers 1 part per million of mercury in seafood to be safe. However, top predator fish such as shark and swordfish can have mercury concentrations over 1 part per million. The FDA recommends no more than one serving a week of these two fish for most people and no more than one serving a month for pregnant or nursing women or those who may become pregnant.[29]

Sounds to me like the "symptoms" caused by mercury exposure can look a lot like most, if not all, autoimmune diseases (have a look at the partial list below) and are certainly suspiciously similar to autism. I believe mercury and metals in general (whether from food, dental fillings, or air pollution) are a major health problem for each

---

29   http://www.medterms.com/script/main/art.asp?articlekey=10991

and every one of us. If they're not the direct cause of a health issue, they may well be a related cause or trigger one.

How can anyone not wonder about links between all the so-called autoimmune diseases and mercury along with other dental metals? Here is a partial list of autoimmune diseases and related conditions:

> active chronic hepatitis, Addison's disease, anti-phospholipid syndrome, atopic allergy, autoimmune atrophic gastritis, achlorhydra, autoimmune celiac disease, Crohn's disease, Cushing's syndrome, dermatomyositis, (Type I) diabetes, discoid lupus, erythematosis, Goodpasture's syndrome, Grave's disease, Hashimoto's thyroiditis, idiopathic adrenal atrophy, idiopathic thrombocytopenia, insulin-dependent diabetes, Lambert-Eaton syndrome, lupoid hepatitis, lymphopenia (some cases), mixed connective tissue disease, multiple sclerosis, pemphigoid, pemphigus vulgaris, pernicious anema, phacogenic uveitis, polyarteritis nodosa, polyglandular auto syndromes, primary biliary cirrhosis, primary sclerosing cholangitis, psoriasis, Raynauds Reiter's syndrome, relapsing polychondritis, rheumatoid arthritis, Schmidt's syndrome, scleroderma — CREST, Sjogren's syndrome, sympathetic ophthalmia, systemic lupus, erythematosis, Takayasu's arteritis, temporal arteritis, thyrotoxicosis, Type B insulin resistance, ulcerative colitis, Wegener's granulomatosis[30]

Just to give you a bit more insight into the mercury issue, following is a section of a paper written by Bernard Windham. The entire paper, along with footnote references, can be found at www.home. earthlink.net/~berniew1/ms.htm. It is rather lengthy and somewhat technical, but a fantastic example of what is available to you and why

---

30 http://www.healinglight.com/autoimmune/types.html

you need to go looking for it as part of taking charge of your health and life.

Mercury from Amalgam Fillings — A Common Cause of MS, ALS, PD, SLE, RA, MCS, AD, etc.

Bernard Windham (Ed.), Chemical Engineer

I. Introduction

Proper functioning of the human body and mind depends on interactions of the brain and CNS using neuronal signaling mechanisms with elaborate metabolic and enzymatic processes and respiration that occurs at the cellular level in the various organs and parts of the body, as controlled by low levels of hormones from the endocrine system. It will be shown that toxic substances, such as mercury that the body is chronically exposed to, accumulate in the brain, pituitary gland, CNS, liver, kidneys, etc. and can damage, inhibit, and cause imbalances at virtually any stage of these various processes at very low levels of exposure, which can have major neurological, immunological, and metabolic effects on an individual.

Mercury is known to be one of the most toxic substances commonly encountered and to be along with lead the toxic substances adversely affecting the largest numbers of people. The main factors determining whether chronic conditions are induced by metals appear to be exposure and genetic susceptibility, which determines individuals' immune sensitivity and ability to detoxify metals. Very low levels of exposure have been found to seriously affect relatively large groups of individuals who are immune sensitive to toxic metals, or have an inability to detoxify metals due to such as deficient sulfoxidation or metallothionein function or other inhibited enzymatic processes related to detoxification or excretion of metals.

As far back as 1996 it was shown that the lesions produced in the myelin sheath of axons in cases of multiple sclerosis were related to excitatory receptors on the primary cells involved called oligodendroglia. The loss of myelin sheath on the nerve fibers characteristic of the disease is due to the death of these oligodendroglial cells at the site of the lesions (called plaques). Further, these studies have shown that the death of these important cells is as a result of excessive exposure to excitotoxins at the site of the lesions. Most of these excitotoxins are secreted from microglial immune cells in the central nervous system. This not only destroys these myelin-producing cells it also breaks down the blood-brain barrier (BBB), allowing excitotoxins in the blood stream to enter the site of damage. Some common exposures that cause such proliferation of such excitotoxins are mercury and aspartame, with additional effects from MSG and methanol. Aspartame and methanol are both in diet drinks and many may drink diet drinks with Chinese food that has MSG.

Mercury and aspartame have been found to be causes of MS, along with other contributing exicitotoxins. It is now known the cause for the destruction of the myelin in the lesions is overactivation of the microglia in the region of the myelin. An enzyme that converts glutamine to glutamate called glutaminase increases tremendously, thereby greatly increasing excitotoxicity. Any dietary excitotoxin can activate the microglia, thereby greatly aggravating the injury. This includes the aspartate in aspartame. The methanol adds to this toxicity as well. Now, the secret to treatment appears to be shutting down, or at least calming down, the microglia.

According to neurologist Dr. RL Blaylock, the good news is that there are supplements and nutrients that calm the microglia — the most potent are: silymarin, curcumin and ibuprophen. Phosphatidylcholine helps re-myelinate the nerve sheaths that are damaged, as does B_{12}, B_6, B_1, vitamin D, folate, vitamin C, natural vitamin E (mixed tocopherols) and L-carnitine. DHA plays a major role in repairing the myelin sheath. Vitamin D may even prevent MS, but it acts as an immune modulator, preventing further damage — the dose is 2000 IU a day. Magnesium, as magnesium malate, is needed in a dose of 500 mg 2X a day. They must avoid all excitotoxins, even natural ones in foods — such as soy, red meats, nuts, mushrooms and tomatoes. Avoid all fluoride and especially all vaccinations since these either inhibit antioxidant enzymes or trigger harmful immune reactions.

It has also been found that the antibiotic minocycline powerfully shuts down the microglia. Dr. Blaylock tried this treatment on a friend of mine who just came down with fulminant MS. He was confined to a wheelchair. I had him placed on minocycline and now, just a few weeks later, he is walking.

The various neurological, immune, and metabolic related diseases discussed together here are diagnosed and labeled clinically based primarily on symptoms, along with tests for some underlying conditions found common in each disease. But each individual will be seen to have their own unique combination of neurological, endocrine, and enzymatic imbalances along with autoimmunities that result in the functional problems that lead to symptoms that are diagnosed as multiple sclerosis (MS) or Amyotropic Lateral Sclerosis (ALS) or Alzheimer's Disease (AD), or Parkinson's Disease (PD), or Systemic Lupus Erythematosus (SLE), rheumatoid arthritis (RA), chronic fatigue syndrome (CFS), or oral lichen planus (OLP), etc. However, a lot of commonality among these factors has been documented, both within specific diseases and among the various diseases discussed here. In MS, an autoimmune T-cell attack on CNS myelin sheath results in demyelinated plaques. Activated T-cells, plasma cells, and macrophages have been found in the demyelinated areas. ALS is a systemic motor neuron disease that affects the corticospinal and corticobulbar tracts, ventral horn motor neurons, and motor cranial nerve nuclei. Approximately 10 percent of ALS cases are of the familial type that has been linked to a mutation of the copper/zinc super oxide dismustase gene (Cu/Zn SOD). The majority of ALS cases are of the sporadic type. There are many toxic substances as well as some common drugs that have been found to be major factors in producing the functional conditions that result in these diseases. However mercury appears to be the most commonly implicated of these, and in particular mercury from amalgam fillings — as will be documented here. For the majority of cases there are now tests to identify the various factors involved in these types of diseases; and once an individual's underlying causative factors have been identified, high success rates at cure or significant improvement are being achieved.

Toxic metals such as mercury, lead, cadmium, etc. have been documented to be neurotoxic, immunotoxic, reproductive/developmental toxins that according to U.S. Government agencies cause adverse health effects and learning disabilities to millions in the U.S. each year, especially children and the elderly. Exposure of humans and animals to toxic metals such as mercury, cadmium, lead, copper, aluminum, arsenic, chromium, manganese, etc. is widespread and in many areas increasing. The U.S. Centers for Disease Control ranks toxic metals as the number one environmental health threat to children. According to an EPA/ATSDR assessment, the toxic metals mercury, lead, and arsenic are the top 3 toxics having the most adverse health effects on the public based on toxicity and current exposure levels in the U.S., with cadmium, nickel and chromium also highly listed.

While there is considerable commonality to the health effects commonly caused by these toxic metals, and effects are cumulative and synergistic in many cases, this paper will concentrate on the health effects of elemental mercury from amalgam fillings. The reason is that the public appears to be generally unaware that considerable scientific evidence supports that mercury is the metal causing the most widespread adverse health effects to the public, and amalgam fillings have been well documented to be the number one source of exposure of mercury to most people, with exposure levels often exceeding Government health guidelines and levels documented to cause adverse health effects. Much of the direct chronic exposure to toxic metals for persons with the autoimmune diseases discussed here appears to be from use of metals in dental work. The most common dental metals that have been documented to be causing widespread adverse health effects are mercury, nickel, palladium, gold, and copper. Although chronic exposure clearly is affecting a much larger population, nickel has been found to be a major factor in many cases of MS and lupus, with palladium having very similar effects to nickel. Likewise chronic exposure to manganese and copper have been implicated in some cases of Parkinson's disease. Another group of toxic substances with widespread exposure that have been demonstrated to generate reactive oxygen species and have positive correlations to some of the diseases discussed here are the organochlorine pesticides. Toxic metals appear to be only one of the factors involved in chronic autoimmune conditions. Pathogens such as viruses, mycoplasma, bacteria and parasites have been found to usually be present and a factor to deal with in treating those with chronic degenerative conditions and weakened immune systems such as MS and other autoimmune conditions.

II. Documentation of High Common Exposures and Accumulation of Mercury in the Brain and Motor Neurons

Amalgam fillings are the largest source of mercury in most people with daily exposures documented to commonly be above government health guidelines. This is due to continuous vaporization of mercury from amalgam in the mouth, along with galvanic currents from mixed metals in the mouth that deposit the mercury in the gums and oral cavity. Due to the high daily mercury exposure and excretion into home and business sewers of those with amalgam, dental amalgam is also the largest source of the high levels of mercury found in all sewers and sewer sludge, and thus according to government studies a significant source of mercury in rivers, lakes, bays, fish, and crops. People also get significant exposure from vaccinations, fish, and dental office vapor.

When amalgam was placed into teeth of monkeys and rats, within one year mercury was found to have accumulated in the brain, trigeminal ganglia, spinal ganglia, kidneys, liver, lungs, hormone glands, and lymph glands. People also commonly get exposures to mercury and other toxic metals such as lead, arsenic, nickel, and aluminum from food, water, and other sources. All of these are highly neurotoxic and are documented to cause neurological damage which can result in chronic neurological conditions over time, as well as ADHD, mood, and behavioral disorders.

Mercury is one of the most toxic substances in existence and is known to bioaccumulate in the body of people and animals that have chronic exposure. Mercury exposure is cumulative and comes primarily from 4 main sources: silver (mercury) dental fillings, food(mainly fish), vaccinations, and occupational exposure. Whereas mercury exposure from fish is primarily methyl mercury and mercury from vaccinations is thimerosal (ethyl mercury), mercury from occupational exposure and dental fillings is primarily from elemental mercury vapor. Developmental and neurological conditions occur at lower levels of exposure from mercury vapor than from inorganic mercury or methyl mercury. Mercury in amalgam fillings, because of its low vapor pressure and galvanic action with other metals in the mouth, has been found to be continuously vaporized and released into the body, and has been found to be directly correlated to the number of amalgam surfaces and the largest source of mercury in the majority of people, typically between 60 and 90% of the total. The level of daily exposure of those with several amalgam fillings commonly exceeds the u.s. epa health guideline for daily mercury exposure of 0.1 ug/kg body weight/day, and the oral mercury level commonly exceeds the mercury MRL of the u.s. atsdr of 0.2 ug/ cubic meter of air. When amalgam fillings are replaced, levels of mercury in the blood, urine, and feces typically rise temporarily but decline between 60 to 85% within 6 to 9 months.

Mercury has been found to accumulate preferentially in the brain, major organs, hormone glands, and primary motor function related areas involved in ALS — such as the brain stem, cerebellum, rhombencephalon, dorsal root ganglia, and anterior horn motor neurons, which enervate the skeletal muscles. Mercury, with exposure either to vapor or organic mercury, tends to accumulate in the glial cells in a similar pattern, and the pattern of deposition is the same as that seen from morphological changes. Though mercury vapor and organic mercury readily cross the blood-brain barrier, mercury has been found to be taken up into neurons of the brain and CNS without having to cross the blood-brain barrier, since mercury has been found to be taken up and transported along nerve axons as well through calcium and sodium channels and along the olfactory path.[31]

Before moving on, I do want to note that Mr. Windham's position on mercury is also discussed on the FDA.GOV website and can at this writing be accessed at the web address as footnoted.[32]

The potential connection between mercury and autism is a long study in and of itself. Given the tendency of mercury to affect unborn children (as noted above), topping off that pre-birth exposure with another potentially near-toxic dose in some vaccinations (children's, flu, or otherwise) is certainly a recipe for disaster.

The accumulation of mercury and other metals or potentially toxic materials in our bodies is a time bomb waiting to be triggered. In my opinion, the growing number of kids with autism and adults with multiple sclerosis and Alzheimer's simply cannot be written off as coincidence.

MERCURY AND ME

There is no doubt in my mind, based on the testing performed on me, and my research, that mercury was a factor contributing to my scary diagnosis. It may have even been the root cause.

Given my scary diagnosis, and my research on mercury, I decided to have my amalgam fillings removed. (I also changed to pots and

---

31 http://www.home.earthlink.net/~berniew1/ms.html
32 http://www.fda.gov/ohrms/dockets/dockets/00n_1665/00N-1665-EC-06.html

pans made of high-quality stainless steel and avoid using aluminum foil.)

I had a series of intravenous chelations and dropped my measurable mercury (measured by a urine test combined with a chelation challenge) from over 120 to 0.46. I regularly detox for heavy metals now using oral chelation and detoxing footpads. (See my website, www.ScaryDiagnosis.com, for details.)

My biological dentist, a concerned, caring, and knowledgeable woman named Dr. Oksana Sawiak, and her staff were a wealth of information and a valuable resource for me. Not only was Dr. Sawiak willing to take the time to discuss my issues in detail, but she also suggested readings and topics that would help educate me about my choices. She understands the potential impact of modern dentistry on the immune system and health in general and is constantly trying to improve her methods to be as safe and effective as possible for her patient — the whole patient, that is.

Her office was equipped with the staff and equipment to do an efficient and effective job of removing my mercury safely while taking the most complete and comprehensive look at my mouth and dental health that I had ever experienced. More and more dentists are catching on to some of these crucial dental issues that may have profound effects on overall health.

Taking the time to find the right dentist may add some additional work to your to-do list, but asking around (try asking at health food stores, chiropractors' offices, and other health and wellness practitioners' offices, in addition to checking the newsletters that are often available free at those locations) is more than worth your time.

Unfortunately, some of these most complete and efficient dentists get less than resounding support from their respective professional organizations or other local dentists. After being worked on by a dentist and staff that are so good, past dental experiences look pretty mediocre to me.

I should add that this more complete and comprehensive approach to dental and oral health was more expensive than the run-of-the-mill offices I had visited in the past. For me, this was a great example of "getting what you pay for." I strongly believe that oral health and dental issues were related, in some significant way, to my scary diagnosis.

WHAT'S HAUNTING DENTISTS

So why is mercury still used in dentistry? Why do many of us have mercury fillings in our mouths? And, by the way, not all fillings containing mercury are silver in color. More recent ones are often white (or almost white, anyway). So why are *any* mercury fillings still around?

Well, just think what would happen if all of a sudden the ADA and CDA admitted that dentists have been poisoning us all these years. The number of lawsuits would be beyond comprehension. The anger and panic would be scary. Dentists, who already have a high suicide rate ... well, you get the idea.

As I was writing that last bit I couldn't help wondering, given the symptoms of mercury toxicity or poisoning, whether there is some kind of mercury connection between mercury and the suicide issue.

No, there will likely be no public confession, no taking of responsibility for the issues surrounding mercury (dental or otherwise) until most or all of those people that had mercury placed in their mouths (or had it injected in a vaccine or ate or breathed it) are dead and gone. It's an accepted fact that mercury is a problem in seafood and fish. But somehow it's fine to stick gobs of it into someone's mouth in the form of a clay-like amalgam that hardens into a lump of silver metal, or leave old ones in there to break down. Go figure.

And mercury is just one of the issues haunting dentistry.

Dentists no doubt mean well and tooth decay was and is an important issue. The business of dentistry still relies on cavities and their prevention or filling as a profitable source of revenue. The fact that materials used to fill cavities can result in some serious problems was certainly not by design.

The newer non-mercury white fillings are often complex plastics. They are thought to be safer. There are lots of different kinds and most are less durable than the old metal ones, which has been one of the arguments for keeping the mercury ones around. Anyone having anything cemented or otherwise inserted into their mouths on a long-term basis should do some research before agreeing to the use of *any* material, metal or plastic.

MERCURY AND YOU

I know, you're probably thinking, "I have a busy life and my dentist is a professional, so why do I have to do any homework or research?"

Because at the end of the day the person hearing and living with that scary diagnosis is you.

Ask your dentist(s) what they're using and what options you may have. Some people are sensitive or allergic to some materials. Having one of these materials used to fill a tooth or make a cap may trigger any number of long-term health issues. The short-term effects may be subtle, but long-term they can wear you down. It's your mouth and your body. You have a right to ask questions and get answers based on the best and most current information.

Proper removal of dental metal is expensive and potentially dangerous, but it's one of those "little" things you can do. Some people have reported getting well almost immediately. For others it is a slower, long-term process. Having mercury removed from their mouths and bodies, and then minimizing additional exposure, seemed important enough to grab their attention. And yes, still others have experienced no obvious results.

But remember this: In all likelihood it took you a very long time to build up mercury and other toxins to the point where you became symptomatic. It's only logical it will take a long time to get rid of the stuff. When our bodies aren't working properly, we may not be able to get rid of it at all. We may have a genetic predisposition. We may need help. But if we don't acknowledge the buildup of mercury, heavy metals, and other toxins as a problem, why would we even think about trying to address them as problems?

In addition to mercury there are lots of other metals used in dentistry that end up in your mouth and body. Some of those metals are part of the amalgam that makes up a mercury-based filling. Others are metals found in various caps or crowns. The metals used in kids' braces can be another area of concern. When you're sick it's important to investigate what is actually in your mouth and when it was put there, and also to take a look back at what used to be in your mouth and question how it may still be affecting you.

Gold is often considered the best dental metal because it's strong and not very reactive. It seems to be best tolerated by the largest number of people. The problem is that pure gold is too soft, so the gold in your mouth is probably an alloy. That means it is mixed with — you guessed it — other stuff including other metals.

I know it seems everything has a downside, and to some extent that's true. That doesn't mean you need to feel and think everything is bad or negative. It does mean it's worth the time and effort to make the best possible choices at any given time. The only way to do that is to be aware of the choices and to understand as well as possible what the pros and cons of each choice are.

By the way, the obvious solution to all this dental and mouth stuff is to take extra special care of your teeth and gums so you don't get stuff drilled and filled into your mouth or need the dreaded root canal to begin with.

It is important to take not only a proactive approach but also a positive one. Whenever we put something into our mouths or bodies that really doesn't belong there, we change everything. To some extent the same holds true for getting stuff removed from our mouths and bodies.

We change the way our entire body works.

Have you ever seen what happens to a stream when a tree falls and blocks just a small part of the flow? Not only does the water flow change to get past the blockage, but downstream the water flows in a new and different way for a fair distance. We often can't tell for a long period of time what will happen downstream as a result of our choices, because time is required to see the full effect. Sometimes the results are startling. There are all kinds of streams and flows in our bodies and most of us have way too many "trees" blocking some of our natural flows. Some of our scary diagnoses are no doubt related to, triggered by, or the direct result of changes made to our bodies.

Here's another important lesson I learned that is well worth spending some time contemplating: We may trigger an effect or result somewhere other than where we intended.

We live in an environment that has changed drastically from almost every perspective since recorded history, so we need to deal with the cumulative issues affecting us today. We may also need to address issues from our individual pasts.

What happened to you as a child or even in the womb (remember mercury and the placenta) may play an important role in your health and wellness, or lack thereof, today.

I never promised you that working on these issues would be easy.

Yes, we need to address the potential problems tooth decay or removal and root canals may cause. But we should be given the opportunity to make choices about how to address those problems based on current and complete information.

There is nothing perfect here on earth so we can only hope to do the best we can.

Do some homework, ask questions, and make the best informed decision you can. It's the best we can do.

ROOT CANALS

Unfortunately I didn't take good enough care of my teeth when I was younger to avoid needing to have root canals later. I thought I had, but the results prove otherwise.

Perhaps my eating and drinking habits affected my teeth more than the same habits would have affected some folks' teeth (back to that genetic predisposition or the "spout" on the teapot). Perhaps, as a result of my lifestyle and personality, my body chemistry made me more susceptible to tooth decay.

In any case, I have four root canals in my mouth and they really have me worried. I am convinced root canals are bad, but the only alternative today seems to be to have the teeth pulled.

There's no way, and I mean no way, I am having something metal implanted in my jaw, and I'm not enthusiastic about a bridge because two of my root canals are rear molars, which means removable bridges. Teeth that may need a root canal can sometimes be saved by treatment with infrared lasers, but it's too late for my four. I have also read recently about injecting ozonated sterile water, but again that's a subject to research rather than a suggestion.

So why I am freaked out about root canals?

Read this from Dr. Mercola's website (this interview may also be found in several other places).

Root Canals Pose Health Threat
An Interview with George Meinig, D.D.S.

Dr. Meinig brings a most curious perspective to an exposé of latent dangers of root canal therapy — fifty years ago he was one of the founders of the American Association of Endodontists (root canal specialists). So he's filled his share of root canals. And when he wasn't filling canals himself, he was teaching the technique to dentists across the country at weekend seminars and clinics. About two years ago, having recently retired, he decided to read all 1174 pages of the detailed research of Dr. Weston Price (D.D.S). Dr. Meinig was startled and shocked. Here was valid documentation of systemic illnesses resulting from latent infections lingering in filled roots. He has since written a book, "Root Canal Cover-Up EXPOSED — Many Illnesses Result," and is devoting himself to radio, TV, and personal appearances before groups in an attempt to blow the whistle and alert the public.

MJ: Please explain what the problem is with root canal therapy.

GM: First, let me note that my book is based on Dr. Weston Price's twenty-five years of careful, impeccable research. He led a 60-man team of researchers whose findings — suppressed until now — rank right up there with the greatest medical discoveries of all time. This is not the usual medical story of a prolonged search for the difficult-to-find causative agent of some devastating disease. Rather, it's the story of how a "cast of millions" (of bacteria) become entrenched inside the structure of teeth and end up causing the largest number of diseases ever traced to a single source.

MJ: What diseases? Can you give us some examples?

GM: Yes, a high percentage of chronic degenerative diseases can originate from root filled teeth. The most frequent were heart and circulatory diseases and he found 16 different causative agents for these. The next most common diseases were those of the joints, arthritis and rheumatism. In third place — but almost tied for second — were diseases of the brain and nervous system. After that, any disease you can name might (and in some cases has) come from root filled teeth.

Let me tell you about the research itself. Dr. Price undertook his investigations in 1900. He continued until 1925, and published his work in two volumes in 1923. In 1915 the National Dental Association (which changed its name a few years later to The American Dental Association) was so impressed with his work that they appointed Dr. Price their first Research Director. His Advisory Board read like a Who's Who in medicine and dentistry for that era. They represented the fields of bacteriology, pathology, rheumatology, surgery, chemistry, and cardiology.

At one point in his writings Dr. Price made this observation: "Dr. Frank Billings (M.D.), probably more than any other American internist, is due credit for the early recognition of the importance of streptococcal focal infections in systemic involvements."

What's really unfortunate here is that very valuable information was covered up and totally buried some 70 years ago by a minority group of autocratic doctors who just didn't believe or couldn't grasp the focal infection theory.

MJ: What is the "focal infection" theory?

GM: This states that germs from a central focal infection — such as teeth, teeth roots, inflamed gum tissues, or maybe tonsils — metastasize to hearts, eyes, lungs, kidneys, or other organs, glands and tissues, establishing new areas of the same infection. Hardly theory any more, this has been proven and demonstrated many times over. It's 100% accepted today. But it was revolutionary thinking during World War I days, and the early 1920's.

Today, both patients and physicians have been "brain washed" to think that infections are less serious because we now have antibiotics. Well, yes and no. In the case of root-filled teeth, the no-longer-living tooth lacks a blood supply to its interior. So circulating antibiotics don't faze the bacteria living there because they can't get at them.

MJ: You're assuming that *all* root-filled teeth harbor bacteria and/or other infective agents?

GM: Yes. No matter what material or technique is used — and this is just as true today — the root filling shrinks minutely, perhaps microscopically. Further and this is key — the bulk of solid appearing teeth, called the dentin, actually consists of miles of tiny tubules. Microscopic organisms lurking in the maze of tubules simply migrate into the interior of the tooth and set up housekeeping. A filled root seems to be a favorite spot to start a new colony.

One of the things that makes this difficult to understand is that large, relatively harmless bacteria common to the mouth, change and adapt to new conditions. They shrink in size to fit the cramped quarters and even learn how to exist (and thrive) on very little food. Those that need oxygen mutate and become able to get along without it. In the process of adaptation these formerly friendly "normal" organisms become pathogenic (capable of producing disease) and more virulent (stronger) and they produce much more potent toxins.

Today's bacteriologists are confirming the discoveries of the Price team of bacteriologists. Both isolated in root canals the same strains of streptococcus, staphylococcus and spirochetes.

MJ: Is everyone who has ever had a root canal filled made ill by it?

GM: No. We believe now that every root canal filling does leak and bacteria do invade the structure. But the variable factor is the strength of the person's immune system. Some healthy people are able to control the germs that escape from their teeth into other areas of the body. We think this happens because their immune system lymphocytes (white blood cells) and other disease fighters aren't constantly compromised by other ailments. In other words, they are able to prevent those new colonies from taking hold in other tissues throughout the body. But over time, most people with root filled teeth do seem to develop some kinds of systemic symptoms they didn't have before.

MJ: It's really difficult to grasp that bacteria are imbedded deep in the structure of seemingly-hard, solid looking teeth.

GM: I know. Physicians and dentists have that same problem, too. You really have to visualize the tooth structure — all of those microscopic tubules running through the dentin. In a healthy tooth, those tubules transport a fluid that carries nourishment to the inside. For perspective, if the tubules of a front single-root tooth were stretched out on the ground they'd stretch for three miles.

A root filled tooth no longer has any fluid circulating through it, but the maze of tubules remains. The anaerobic bacteria that live there seem remarkably safe from antibiotics. The bacteria can migrate out into surrounding tissue where they can "hitch hike" to other locations in the body via the bloodstream. The new location can be any organ or gland or tissue, and the new colony will be the next focus of infection in a body plagued by recurrent or chronic infections.

All of the "building up" done to try to enhance the patient's ability to fight infections — to strengthen their immune system — is only a holding action. Many patients won't be well until the source of infection — the root canal tooth — is removed.

MJ: I don't doubt what you're saying, but can you tell us more about how Dr. Price could be sure that arthritis or other systemic conditions and illnesses really originated in the teeth — or in a single tooth?

GM: Yes. Many investigations start with the researcher just being curious about something — and then being scientifically careful enough to discover an answer, and then prove it's so, many times over. Dr. Price's first case is very well documented. He removed an infected tooth from a woman who suffered from severe arthritis. As soon as he finished with the patient, he implanted the tooth beneath the skin of a healthy rabbit. Within 48 hours the rabbit was crippled with arthritis.

Further, once the tooth was removed the patient's arthritis improved dramatically. This clearly suggested that the presence of the infected tooth was a causative agent for both that patient's and the rabbit's arthritis.

(Editor's Note: Here's the story of that first patient from Dr. Meinig's book.)

(Dr. Price) had a sense that, even when (root canal therapy) appeared successful, teeth containing root fillings remained infected. That thought kept preying on his mind, haunting him each time a patient consulted him for relief from some severe debilitating disease for which the medical profession could find no answer. Then one day while treating a woman who had been confined to a wheelchair for six years from severe arthritis, he recalled how bacterial cultures were taken from patients who were ill and then inoculated into animals in an effort to reproduce the disease and test the effectiveness of drugs on the disease.

With this thought in mind, although her (root filled) tooth looked fine, he advised this arthritic patient to have it extracted. He told her he was going to find out what it was about this root filled tooth that was responsible for her suffering. All dentists know that sometimes arthritis and other illnesses clear up if bad teeth are extracted. However, in this case, all of her teeth appeared in satisfactory condition and the one containing this root canal filling showed no evidence or symptoms of infection. Besides, it looked normal on x-ray pictures.

Immediately after Dr. Price extracted the tooth he dismissed the patient and embedded her tooth under the skin of a rabbit. In two days the rabbit developed the same kind of crippling arthritis as the patient — and in ten days it died.

The patient made a successful recovery after the tooth's removal. She could then walk without a cane and could even do fine needlework again. That success led Dr. Price to advise other patients, afflicted with a wide variety of treatment defying illnesses, to have any root filled teeth out.

In the years that followed, he repeated this procedure many hundreds of times. He later implanted only a portion of the tooth to see if that produced the same results. It did. He then dried the tooth, ground it into powder and injected a tiny bit into several rabbits. Same results, this time producing the same symptoms in multiple animals.

Dr. Price eventually grew cultures of the bacteria and injected them into the animals. Then he went a step further. He put the solution containing the bacteria through a filter small enough to catch the bacteria. So when he injected the resulting liquid it was free of any infecting bacteria. Did the test animals develop the illness? Yes. The only explanation was that the liquid had to contain toxins from the bacteria, and the toxins were also capable of causing disease.

Dr. Price became curious about which was the more potent infective agent, the bacteria or the toxin. He repeated that last experiment, injecting half the animals with the toxin-containing liquid and half of them with the bacteria from the filter. Both groups became ill, but the group injected with the toxins got sicker and died sooner than the bacteria injected animals.

MJ: That's amazing. Did the rabbits always develop the same disease the patient had?

GM: Mostly, yes. If the patient had heart disease the rabbit got heart disease. If the patient had kidney disease the rabbit got kidney disease, and so on. Only occasionally did a rabbit develop a different disease — and then the pathology would be quite similar, in a different location.

MJ: If extraction proves necessary for anyone reading this, do you want to summarize what's special about the extraction technique?

GM: Just pulling the tooth is not enough when removal proves necessary. Dr. Price found bacteria in the tissues and bone just adjacent to the tooth's root. So we now recommend slow-speed drilling with a burr, to remove one millimeter of the entire bony socket. The purpose is to remove the periodontal ligament (which is always infected with toxins produced by streptococcus bacteria living in the dentin tubules) and the first millimeter of bone that lines the socket (which is usually infected).

There's a whole protocol involved, including irrigating with sterile saline to assure removal of the contaminated bone chips, and treating the socket to stimulate and encourage infection-free healing. I describe the procedure in detail, step by step, in my book [pages 185 and 186].

MJ: Perhaps we should back up and talk about oral health — to *prevent* needing an extraction. Caries or inflamed gums seem much more common than root canals. Do they pose any threat?

GM: Yes, they absolutely do. But let me point out that we can't talk about oral health apart from total health. The problem is that patients and dentists alike haven't come around to seeing that dental caries reflect systemic — meaning "whole body" — illness. Dentists have learned to restore teeth so expertly that both they and their patients have come to regard tooth decay as a trivial matter. It isn't.

Small cavities too often become big cavities. Big cavities too often lead to further destruction and the eventual need for root canal treatment.

MJ: Then talk to us about prevention.

GM: The only scientific way to prevent tooth decay is through diet and nutrition. Dr. Ralph Steinman did some outstanding, landmark research at Loma Linda University. He injected a glucose solution into mice — into their bodies, so the glucose didn't even touch their teeth. Then he observed the teeth for any changes. What he found was truly astonishing. The glucose reversed the normal flow of fluid in the dentin tubules, resulting in all of the test animals developing severe tooth decay. Dr. Steinman demonstrated dramatically what I said a minute ago: Dental caries reflect systemic illness.

Let's take a closer look to see how this might happen. Once a tooth gets infected and the cavity gets into the nerve and blood vessels, bacteria find their way into those tiny tubules of the dentin. Then no matter what we do by way of treatment, we're never going to completely eradicate the bacteria hiding in the miles of tubules. In time the bacteria can migrate through lateral canals into the surrounding bony socket that supports the tooth. Now the host not only has a cavity in a tooth, plus an underlying infection of supporting tissue to deal with, but the bacteria also exude potent systemic toxins. These toxins circulate throughout the body triggering activity by the immune system — and probably causing the host to feel less well. This host response can vary from just dragging around and feeling less energetic, to overt illness — of almost any kind. Certainly, such a person will be more vulnerable to whatever "bugs" are going around, because his/her body is already under constant challenge and the immune system continues to be "turned on" by either the infective agent or its toxins — or both.

MJ: What a fascinating concept. Can you tell us more about the protective nutrition you mentioned?

GM: Yes. Dr. Price traveled all over the world doing his research on primitive peoples who still lived in their native ways. He found fourteen cultural pockets scattered all over the globe where the natives had no access to "civilization" — and ate no refined foods.

Dr. Price studied their diets carefully. He found they varied greatly, but the one thing they had in common was that they ate whole, unrefined foods. With absolutely no access to tooth brushes, floss, fluoridated water or tooth paste, the primitive peoples studied were almost 100% free of tooth decay. Further — and not unrelated — they were also almost 100% free of all the degenerative diseases we suffer — problems with the heart, lungs, kidneys, liver, joints, skin (allergies), and the whole gamut of illnesses that plague mankind. No one food proved to be magic as a preventive food. I believe we can thrive best by eating a wide variety of whole foods.

MJ: Amazing. So by "diet and nutrition" for oral (and total) health you meant eating a pretty basic diet of whole foods?

GM: Exactly. And no sugar or white flour. These are (and always have been) the first culprits. Tragically, when the primitives were introduced to sugar and white flour their superior level of health deteriorated rapidly. This has been demonstrated time and again. During the last sixty or more years we have added in increasing amounts, highly refined and fabricated cereals and boxed mixes of all kinds, soft drinks, refined vegetable oils and a whole host of other foodless "foods." It is also during those same years that we as a nation have installed more and more root canal fillings — and degenerative diseases have become rampant. I believe — and Dr. Price certainly proved to my satisfaction — that these simultaneous factors are *not* coincidences.

MJ: I certainly understand what you are saying. But I'm still a little shocked to talk with a dentist who doesn't stress oral hygiene.

GM: Well, I'm not against oral hygiene. Of course, hygiene practices are preventive, and help minimize the destructive effect of our "civilized," refined diet. But the real issue is still diet. The natives Dr. Price tracked down and studied weren't free of cavities, inflamed gums, and degenerative diseases because they had better tooth brushes.

It's so easy to lose sight of the significance of what Dr. Price discovered. We tend to sweep it under the rug — we'd actually prefer to hear that if we would just brush better, longer, or more often, we too could be free of dental problems.

Certainly, part of the purpose of my book is to stimulate dental research into finding a way to sterilize dentin tubules. Only then can dentists really learn to save teeth for a lifetime. But the bottom line remains: A primitive diet of whole unrefined foods is the only thing that has been found to actually prevent both tooth decay and degenerative diseases.[33]

---

33   http://www.mercola.com/article/dental/rootcanal/root_canals.htm#

I'm guessing if you have any root canals and especially if you have heard a scary diagnosis, you're a bit worried, too.

Again, diet, especially sugar and white flour, is a recurring theme and an important link to ill health. I'd add pop (soda) and artificial sweeteners to that list.

There does appear to be some hope that using lasers and a material called Biocalex or Biodent makes a more effective root filler, but of course there are folks on both the pro and con sides of these procedures as well.

Please do some Internet searching because this kind of information changes very quickly. I am hoping by the time you read this I will have found an option that makes sense to me for dealing with my own four root canals.

ELEVEN

ADJUSTING YOUR LIFESTYLE

> When you have to make a choice and don't make it,
> that is in itself a choice.
> — WILLIAM JAMES

DIET, GETTING BETTER sleep, exercising—it's amazing how important these can be in helping you take charge of your health and life, no matter what your scary diagnosis.

YOUR DIET

General Pointers

Fruits and vegetables, whole grains, drug-free meats, and moderate amounts of fish (limiting shellfish) all make sense, whether you're healthy or not. Some of us are sensitive to particular foods or beverages, and these should be identified and avoided. One of the best ways I've found to identify things to avoid is through applied kinesiology (AK), or muscle testing. As described above, this procedure tests for sensitivities in a non-intrusive manner and with pretty consistent results using groups of muscles and their responses to stimuli. Some chiropractors are trained in AK. It's becoming more mainstream and is used by some allopathic doctors. It has even been used by a doctor repeatedly on the *Doctor Phil Show.*

Blood tests, urine tests, and scratch tests, along with testing of hair samples, are also available for identifying a wide range of sensitivities and allergies, including foods, chemicals found in your everyday environment, molds, and a great many other things. No doubt many of these tests are quite good. I prefer AK for regular use because it's easy, non-invasive, and economical. That last characteristic is important because things may change often in your body and personal environment and as a result it's best to be tested on a fairly regular basis.

My good friend and chiropractor Dr. Brian Smuk runs a nutritional testing clinic. He offers exactly the kind of programs that give clients the information they need to make smart nutritional and lifestyle decisions. It's a great service that has been, and continues to be, a huge help to me. No doubt this kind of clinic will be more and more common as time goes on. (More information about this and other resources may be found on my website, www.Scary Diagnosis.com.)

Eliminating refined sugar and wheat from your diet (minimizing processed foods) and replacing them with whole grains, eliminating carbonated beverages, and especially eliminating artificial sweeteners, are musts if you're ill or looking to prevent illness. Do the research and decide for yourself, but the arguments, especially concerning most artificial sweeteners, are scary and compelling.

Fish is good but many have high levels of toxic metals and chemicals. Although I love shellfish, I avoid them almost completely now. I eat fish and supplement this part of my diet with mercury-free cod liver or fish oils. They are important and worth learning about for almost all scary diagnoses. Fish oils help reduce cholesterol and have a positive impact on almost every organ and illness. Fish oils are a bigger deal to date in Europe and are often recommended to heart patients, nursing mothers, and critically ill patients.

The more mature among us will remember the dreaded daily spoonful of cod liver oil (before my time). We laugh about it now, but our parents and grandparents may just have known what they were doing.

Interest in organic food is big and will only get bigger. All kinds of chemicals, including pesticides, herbicides, hormones, and anti-biotics, are difficult if not impossible to wash off or out of food, so it's best to buy food and water not exposed to them in the first place. I no longer use herbicides or pesticides around my house.

If possible, get food from local farmers or farmers' markets, or grow some of your own food. In response to growing demand, many "local" farmers are starting to farm without chemicals and minimiz-ing or eliminating the use of many drugs. You will often pay more, but it's worth eliminating as many potentially harmful variables as possible, especially when your body is already weak. I believe that for people with a scary diagnosis, organic, drug-free, and range-fed (free-range, grass-fed) are best.

Processed food is convenient but may put serious pressure on what is often an already overtaxed body and immune system. I'm not talking just about fast food but about anything canned, bottled, or boxed and enhanced with chemicals for taste, color, consistency, or "freshness."

It amazes me that often one of the last things people are willing to address when ill is what they eat and drink. They may read that some sweeteners are linked directly to their condition or that refined sugar does nothing good for them at all. Yet they consider having an operation or undergoing serious treatments before doing something as simple as changing these food and drink variables. Perhaps if more doctors and the media got behind some of what I consider simple common sense precautions, more folks would err on the side of caution.

Just for the record, it also amazes me that good, personalized nutrition is not one of the first things doctors ask about and recommend to us (even through referral). I'm hoping this issue becomes a part of every doctor's approach to helping patients manage a scary diagnosis.

Try to eat chemical-free fresh meat and produce as much as possible. As with all these issues, some argue we should eat lots of raw stuff and others say slightly steamed or baked is best. In general, meat should be thoroughly cooked. Some veggies I eat raw, others lightly cooked. Nutrition is becoming a huge business and there are so many differing opinions and specialty diets that figuring out what's best for you is certainly a challenge.

Here's an example: Is coffee good or bad for you?

If you research it you'll find some say yea — for example, a Japanese study reports coffee may help prevent liver cancer — and some say nay — a Greek study says it appears to increase the risk of heart disease. I don't know, but I don't drink it anymore. I went through a noticeable withdrawal when I eliminated almost all caffeine from my diet (I do drink green tea and eat a bit of dark chocolate). That alone convinced me to stay away from it, and today I don't miss it a bit. Good or bad, it's one less thing for me to worry about.

If you choose to eliminate something from your diet, do it in small, incremental steps. Going cold turkey can be a shock to the system. Even if the end result is good, you should be as kind to your body as possible. After all, your diagnosis may already be putting a considerable strain on your system.

All that said, stressing over not eating something can be far worse for you than eating what you're stressing over to begin with. Attitude is a big part of dealing with a scary diagnosis. Treating yourself occasionally to something you really want will help you keep things positive. I'm not talking about eating nuts if you're allergic to them, but the odd piece of chocolate as opposed to the entire box is fine.

In fact, I had a couple of pieces a few minutes ago. Chocolate is one of those things that may be good for people in general (it seems to hit the news pretty regularly), but a problem for specific illnesses or conditions. I remember reading a comment that people with MS shouldn't be eating it, as it is considered a possible allergen and can result in inflammation and attacks. MSers are urged by some to eliminate potential allergens from their diets and reintroduce them one at a time, if so desired, monitoring any reactions.

There is something to be said for enjoying life (even though that definition is different and changes over time for most of us). Sometimes eating or drinking things we know are not good long-term lifts us up by satisfying our cravings and allowing us to feel the freedom associated with making those choices. Common sense needs to prevail on this one.

My wife and I try to eat and drink right 80% of the time. When we really want something we think we shouldn't have, we indulge ourselves. Over time we have lost our taste for some of the bad stuff we ate and drank and have these things rarely if at all. It is interesting that sometimes we feel good about having indulged, while other times we end up realizing it was the thought of eating or drinking something more than the activity itself that was important to us.

Water

We all know we're made up mostly of water. Let's call it two-thirds to keep it simple. We've got two main systems that allow fluid to flow around in us. Blood is one and lymph the other. Since lymph doesn't get mentioned as often as it should, here's a definition for you:

Lymph

1. A clear, watery, sometimes faintly yellowish fluid derived from body tissues that contains white blood cells and circulates throughout the lymphatic system, returning to the venous bloodstream through the thoracic duct. Lymph acts to remove bacteria and certain proteins from the tissues, transport fat from the small intestine, and supply mature lymphocytes to the blood.
2. *Archaic.* A spring or stream of pure, clear water.[34]

Right off you can see the importance of what lymph does, such as removing bacteria and transporting fat, which are a big part of getting and staying healthy and fit.

I like the last bit of the definition, which talks about a "spring or stream of pure, clear water." For most of us, our lymph is loaded with junk, doesn't move around like it should, and is therefore another source of bad stuff for us to marinate in. Yes, this is a gross over-simplification, and actually just plain gross, but bottom line, it's about right.

The best I can tell, the two most important things you can do for your health and to help your body when it's sick are to drink lots of water (not any old fluid) and get some exercise. Get that lymph moving. Get your blood flowing.

---

34 http://www.answers.com/topic/lymph

Most of us know we need to drink "plenty of fluids" when we're sick. We've heard that forever. Actually, we need to drink plenty of fluids all the time, particularly water.

Hang on a minute — I'm going to get myself a glass of water right now while I'm thinking about it. Why don't you do the same?

I have read all kinds of recommendations regarding the amounts and kinds of fluid we should be drinking. The amounts can range from six or eight cups a day to gallons. But the fluid of preference is good, clean water.

It's not only about how much you drink but what you drink and when you drink it. Apparently, in order for our bodies to make the best use of all this water, there is a limit to how much we should drink at any one time. The most sensible thing I've read is to drink at least four ounces of water an hour, every hour you're awake, if possible. If you feel thirsty, it's too late — you're already dehydrated. If you're exercising or sweating, you need more. By drinking water in reasonable amounts throughout the day, you're constantly hydrating yourself. If it's too much, you just pass it.

It's also best to drink water before a meal but not during or right after a meal, since you don't want to dilute or wash away the stuff that's helping you digest your food. I have read more than once to wait an hour before drinking after a meal. I wonder if that's somehow tied to the old "wait an hour before swimming after a meal" advice.

Don't let me or anyone else decide how much you drink and when you drink it. Do a bit of research and come up with a plan for yourself. Try different amounts and different times. Pay attention to which process helps you feel best.

Most experts promoting the drinking of more fluids recommend just plain water.

This makes sense because *all* of the other stuff we may like to include in our fluid intake has something else other than water in it or it wouldn't be other stuff.

If it is a processed drink containing some "juices," and certainly if it contains pop (or soda depending on where you grew up), all kinds of other things may be included, such as chemicals, preservatives, colorings, refined sugar, or artificial sweeteners. Any of this can be bad for you or make your body work way harder than it should have to for the water part it craves and requires.

Sure, I'd like to include beer, wine, and coffee on the list, but these tend to dehydrate us. What we really need is plain old water. It's easy for the body to use, doesn't make the body work harder than it needs to, and is essential for achieving and maintaining any kind of health.

Whether your doctor agrees or not, we have likely accumulated in our bodies toxic or near-toxic levels of one thing or another, and water helps you move some of this stuff along and out. Water intake may not be enough on its own, but it is a crucial part of any effort to cleanse and detox. You want to dilute the stuff you may be marinating yourself in, and get rid of it.

Here's a little tip: Create some kind of easy system to help you remember to drink water often. Otherwise it can be too easy to forget to drink regularly and you end up drinking a lot at once if at all. Always have a full glass of water sitting next to you (where you can see it all the time). This will encourage you to sip it regularly.

Till now I've been talking about good old plain water, but apparently there's no such thing anymore.

Some people fanatically support drinking spring water, others recommend filtered water, ionized water, ozonated water, tap water, or distilled water. No doubt this list is nowhere close to being complete.

In the early days after my diagnosis, I bought a distiller and was drinking only distilled water for a time. I wanted to make sure there was absolutely nothing in the water I drank — meaning no chemicals, bacteria, etc. Another reason was I was unsure about the plastic some water comes in. Distilled water is made by boiling water and capturing the steam. The steam cools back to a liquid and is collected so you have only the pure water left. Any chemicals, minerals, or impurities are vaporized or left in the boiler. Just for your information, a small amount of a brownish liquid was often left in the "boiler" unit, showing what was in my tap water before I distilled it. Quite frankly, it was gross.

After about six months of drinking distilled water only, I read repeatedly that this was not healthy long-term, although short-term it may be a very good idea. The argument was that distilled water tended to leach out too many minerals needed by our bodies over time.

I also read that spring water could be unreliable. This was based not only on the quality of the source but also on how long it was stored, how the bottles were cleaned, and what the bottles were made of. Some materials used to make bottles leach or leak some of the bottle ingredients into the water over time. When you drink the water, you are also drinking some of the bottle and/or the solvents used to clean it. Occasionally you'll read about these issues in the news. Several of the big players in North America and Europe have had massive recalls of bottled water products. For more information, type "bottled water recalls" into one of your search engines.

Filtered water seemed to get pretty good reviews, depending on the source, the filter, and the age of the filter. Some recommend using ultraviolet light to kill off "living" stuff as part of the filtering process.

There were basically upsides and downsides to each and every kind, type, and brand of water I researched. Water, one of the fundamental ingredients of life, one of the simplest things we can consume regularly to promote and maintain our health and wellness, turned out to be one of the toughest things to pin down.

Water, water everywhere, but what the heck do I drink?

My solution was to drink all of them, except processed tap water, because I believe the chlorine and fluoride used in most municipal water has far more potential health issues than benefits. Here are some facts. Have a read and decide for yourself.

Chlorine (from the Greek language *Chloros*, meaning "pale green"), is the chemical element with atomic number 17 and symbol Cl. It is a halogen, found in the periodic table in group 17. As the chloride ion, which is part of common salt and other compounds, it is abundant in nature and necessary to most forms of life, including the human body. As chlorine gas, it is greenish yellow, is two and one half times as heavy as air, has an intensely disagreeable suffocating odor, and is exceedingly poisonous. In its liquid and solid form it is a powerful oxidizing, bleaching, and disinfecting agent.

Applications
Chlorine is an important chemical for some processes of water purification, in disinfectants, and in bleach. Ozone can also be used for killing bacteria, and is preferred by many municipal drinking water systems because ozone does not

form organochlorine compounds and does not remain in the water after treatment.

Chlorine is also used widely in the manufacture of many everyday items.

*   Used (in the form of hypochlorous acid) to kill bacteria and other microbes from drinking water supplies and swimming pools. Even small water supplies are now routinely chlorinated.
*   Used widely in paper product production, antiseptic, dyestuffs, food, insecticides, paints, petroleum products, plastics, medicines, textiles, solvents, and many other consumer products.

Organic chemistry uses this element extensively as an oxidizing agent and in substitution because chlorine often imparts many desired properties in an organic compound when it is substituted for hydrogen (as in synthetic rubber production).

Other uses are in the production of chlorates, chloroform, carbon tetrachloride, and in the bromine extraction.[35]

Fluorides and Human Health

Higher concentrations

In high concentrations, **fluoride compounds** are toxic. In mice, a "semilethal dose" is estimated to be 184 milligrams of stannous fluoride per kilogram of body mass. Fatalities have been reported in some human individuals at doses as low as 71 mg/kg of sodium fluoride. Symptoms of acute toxicity have been reported to occur in rodents at chronic doses as low as 1 mg/kg.

When ingested directly, fluoride compounds are readily absorbed by the intestines. Over time, the compound is

---

35 http://en.wikipedia.org/wiki/Chlorine

excreted through the urine, and the half life for concentration of fluorine compounds is on an order of hours. Implied is that fluoride is taken out of circulation by the body and trace amounts bound in bone. Urine tests are a good indication of high exposure to fluoride compounds in the recent past.

Skin or eye contact with many fluoride compounds in high concentrations is dangerous. In case of accidental swallowing, milk, calcium carbonate, or milk of magnesia is given to slow absorption. Eye or skin contact is treated by removing any contaminated clothing and flushing with water.

Low concentrations
Fluoride is best known for its use in small quantities to help reduce dental caries (cavity) frequency in teeth.

Fluoride compounds, usually calcium fluoride, are naturally found in low concentration in drinking water and some foods, such as tea. The ocean itself has an average concentration of 1.3 ppm (parts per million). Fluoride ions replace hydroxide ions in calcium hydroxyapatite, $Ca_5[(PO_4)_3OH]$, in teeth, forming calcium fluoroapatite, $Ca_5[(PO_4)_3F]$, which is more chemically stable and dissolves at a pH of 4.5, compared to 5.5 pH for calcium hydroxyapatite. This is generally believed to lead to fewer cavities, since stronger acids are needed to attack the tooth enamel. In 1951, Joseph C. Muhler and Harry G. Day of Indiana University Bloomington reported their research results on stannous fluoride as a tooth decay preventive and the university first sold the technology to Procter & Gamble to use in Crest toothpaste.

The widely accepted adverse effect of low concentration fluoridation at this time is fluorosis. It is a condition caused by "excessive" intake of fluorine compounds over an extended period of time, and can cause yellowing of teeth, hypothyroidism, or brittling of bones and teeth. The definition of "excessive" in the context of fluorosis falls on the order of parts per million and is *generally* accepted to mean significantly higher than the 0.7 to 1.2 ppm amounts recommended for fluoridated water. However, dosage is crucial to adverse effects, and therefore, what concentration is problematic will depend on the amount of fluoride ingested, how much is absorbed, and the weight of the person ingesting it. For this reason, many doctors have advised against using fluoridated water to make up formula for infants. However, this may be more so due to the chemical interaction of fluoride with the calcium in the formula producing CaF_2 which will precipitate out of the body within the stool of the infant, thereby decreasing its absorption. People with kidney problems, or those on dialysis, are also advised not to ingest fluoridated water.

Less widely accepted adverse effects of low concentration fluoridation concern harms that are more systemic in nature. For example, recent research found a significant correlation between degree of pineal gland calcification, and degree of fluoride deposition in this gland. Others believe these low concentrations are causally associated with widespread thyroid disorders; still others believe that cancer may be implicated. However, as of the present, systemic harm arising from low concentration fluoridation remains unknown.[36]

You can make your own decisions about drinking water containing chlorine or fluoride. I avoid them because I have enough problems as it is.

Many believe fluoride has proven itself as a cavity fighter and is good for teeth. Others aren't so sure. The important issue here is how fluoride affects the rest of your body. It turns out it can harm you right down to the cellular level as in fluorosis, noted in the

36 http://en.wikipedia.org/wiki/Floride

above quote. The Canadian Dental Association used to recommend fluoride drops for kids. Not any more.

What may be good for your teeth, a "hard" part of your body that is mostly calcium, phosphorus, and other mineral salts, may not be good for your kidneys, liver, stomach, etc. Make sure you know the *whole* story and make decisions based on what's affecting you most.

Today I mostly drink alkaline water, sometimes referred to as ionized water, which I treat myself. The unit I use has a great filter on it and ionizes water into its acid and alkaline (basic) components.

Alkaline water is gaining momentum in the world of water and health. Some think it's nonsense. Others think it's an important component of good health. The argument is that most of us are too acidic and that many of the things we drink (including distilled water and water filtered by reverse osmosis) tend to make the problem worse. Some feel many of the causes or triggers of disease don't do well in an alkaline environment but tend to thrive in an acidic one. For additional reading on this subject, just put "alkaline water and cancer" (or any illness) into any search engine.

I have limited personal experience with ionized water, but some of the arguments for its use sound sensible to me. I have read some strong arguments against the scientific premise behind its use, but there is mounting anecdotal evidence that there may be something to it. Given my LDN experience (see chapter nine), I tend to pay more and more attention to anecdotal evidence.

It's not easy to tell whether any one particular thing like alkaline water is "working." Because our bodies are complex systems, it's next to impossible to isolate and quantify the effects of a single input (water).

I plan to give it a good look and hope to let you know what I think down the road. Perhaps you should give it a good look, too.

Ozonated water can be another controversial topic, one that requires exploration on your own. Ozone is used to "clean" bottles and treat water. It is also promoted as a healing drink when the water is consumed immediately after it is ozonated.

I have no direct experience with ozone, but its water- and health-related uses make it worth a look. I wanted to mention it because I have come across it a number of times and the potential alternative uses of it are very diverse. Some of the medicinal claims are extraordinary and it's getting more noticeable because it's appearing on the label of some popular brands of water.

Salt

Just a pinch of information on salt. Not salt water or table salt, but natural sea salt. Sea salt that has had nothing added and a minimum of processing.

Salt is essential to life and health. I believe, based on my research, that it has gotten a bad rap, even with respect to blood pressure (we're talking real sea salt here).

Take some time to research salt on the Internet. I believe you'll be surprised — no, shocked — by some of what you find. Dr. Mercola makes some interesting points as a place to start, at www.Mercola. com (Himalayan Salt), and http://www.curezone.com/foods/salt cure.asp covers sea salt in some detail. Here are the benefits of salt, from Mercola.com:

1. Regulating the water content throughout your body.
2. Balancing excess acidity from your cells, particularly your brain cells.
3. Balancing your blood sugar levels and helping to reduce your aging rate.
4. Assisting in the generation of hydroelectric energy in cells in your body.

5. Absorption of food particles through your intestinal tract.
6. Help in clearing mucus plugs and phlegm from your lungs — particularly useful in asthma and cystic fibrosis.
7. Acts as a strong natural antihistamine and helps clear up congestion in your sinuses
8. Prevention of muscle cramps.
9. Making the structure of your bones firm — osteoporosis can occur when your body needs more salt and takes it from your bones.
10. Regulating your sleep — it is a natural hypnotic.
11. Maintaining your libido.
12. Preventing varicose veins and spider veins on your legs and thighs.
13. Stabilizing irregular heartbeats — in conjunction with water it is actually essential for the regulation of your blood pressure.[37]

Salt is a multitasker. It helps us retain proper fluid levels in our bodies and has an impact on the way our body works, right down to the cellular level. It helps with the transmission of electrical impulses, which are what our nerves are all about. There is a significant amount of controversy over which salt, how much, and why. My guess is limiting processed table salt is a good thing. Increasing high-quality sea salt in your diet makes compelling sense, especially when you're ill.

Milk
Of the many things I expect to take grief for in this book, the subject of milk may top the list. I'm going to keep this short and simple and ask you to do your own research and come to your own conclusions. Please remember, my comments on these topics are not meant to be definitive or complete. They are presented merely to start you off on

---

37 http://www.mercola.com/forms/salt.htm

your own research by highlighting issues I found to be significant when doing my research.

Drinking processed cow's milk doesn't make sense to me, and there's plenty of information that brings into question the value of its promotion and use. Cows are typically pumped full of growth hormones and antibiotics that may show up in their milk. Unprocessed cow's milk makes a bit more sense, but for most of us it is just not feasible because it needs to be very fresh and can be prone to contamination.

Goat's milk and products made from it, such as yogurt and kefir, seem far better choices for lots of reasons, including being higher in some stuff like niacin, and the fact that its protein is reportedly easier to digest than cow's milk. No, I don't raise goats or hold stock in World Goat Domination Inc. Do the research and decide for yourself.

Be sure to conduct your search on milk (and milk products) by adding keywords in your search engine, especially as they pertain to your condition. Please, no cards, emails, or letters — your position on milk is up to you and mine is up to me. I avoid all milk and most cow milk products.

Just do some serious research and reading before thinking you understand all the related health issues, including calcium, allergies, lactose intolerance, etc. I was taught way back in school that cow's milk was the "perfect food." I'm guessing that's absolutely correct, if you happen to be a baby cow.

Fresh juice

I'm a real fan of fresh juice, particularly the kind you make at home out of well-scrubbed organic fruits and vegetables and run through a serious juicer. Unfortunately, like most people, I don't make the time to go buy the stuff, clean it, juice it, and drink it nearly as often as I should or would like to.

Juicing is an excellent way to supplement your diet in a really healthy fashion. I urge everyone to look into it and make an effort to juice regularly. I believe it can be a major plus for anyone in a weakened or otherwise compromised position health-wise.

Who doesn't know someone with cancer? Between my wife's two bouts of it and the loss of some close friends, I certainly have. Cancer is a common fear throughout our society. There are tons of people with all kinds of information and personal stories available through articles, books, tapes, and websites. Lorraine Day, a medical doctor, has some material out on her personal experiences with cancer. My wife has two of her tapes, one of which is called *Cancer Doesn't Scare Me Anymore*. Juicing is something she vigorously promotes.

The following is a brief biography from Dr. Day's website:

Dr. Day is an internationally acclaimed orthopedic trauma surgeon and best selling author who was for 15 years on the faculty of the University of California, San Francisco, School of Medicine as Associate Professor and Vice Chairman of the Department of Orthopedics. She was also Chief of Orthopedic Surgery at San Francisco General Hospital and is recognized worldwide as an AIDS expert.

She has been invited to lecture extensively throughout the U.S. and the world and has appeared on numerous radio and television shows including *60 minutes, Nightline, CNN Crossfire, Oprah Winfrey, Larry King Live, The 700 Club, John Ankerberg Show, USA Radio Network, Art Bell Radio Show*, Three Angels Broadcasting Network and Trinity Broadcasting Network.[38]

Dr. Day's story is compelling, and her position on medicine, health, and wellness is enlightened and enlightening, especially given her

---

38   http://www.drday.com/

impeccable medical background. She has been attacked repeatedly in print but has stayed the course and even taken the time to respond to some of the abuses she's been subjected to.

I have no doubt you'll find her personal treatment choices surprising and her position on the politics and business of medicine both disturbing and fascinating. I believe she and some of the issues surrounding her give all kinds of credibility to my core message. You need to be fully informed about and in charge of your own health options.

Turn those search engines on and do some reading so you can decide for yourself. Her site as of this writing is www.drday.com.

Recently I started taking a nutritional supplement that's supposed to be equivalent to fresh organic juices in a pill. I felt the literature on the product was impressive, but I haven't used it long enough to mention it by name here. Several products claim to reproduce the effects of juicing. If you're really ill, drink the real thing for as long as you can. For updated information on my experiences with the juice pill, check my website, www.ScaryDiagnosis.com.

BREATHING

Since most of us don't give much thought to breathing, and because breathing can have such a major impact on our health, let's take a look at it.

You may think I'm stating the obvious, but most of us don't breathe properly or understand how to help ourselves by focusing on our breathing.

Most of us breathe too fast and too shallow, which, according to a lot of research I've read, is not good for digestion or health in general. Breathing can have an impact on all kinds of things and should be looked into by anyone focused on health, especially those who are already ill. Please take the time to learn about proper "belly" breathing. It is simple and easy to take action on, and will impact your health over time. Since most scary diagnoses have waiting and stress in common, no doubt you'll have plenty of time to work on proper breathing.

And smoking? Forget about It.

Okay, there is simply no way to mention breathing without talking about smoking tobacco products. Talk about toxic! Do a search or just read the warning on the packaging.

It amazes me that people can buy and smoke cigarettes, choosing to poison themselves and those around them and subject their bodies to all kinds of potential health problems clearly related to the use of tobacco, and then expect us to "pay the bill" (in so many ways). Smokers are directly or indirectly a major cause if not *the* major cause of the overloading and overburdening of our healthcare systems. Alcohol abuse is certainly right up there, as well. Meanwhile, people with a terminal or degenerative disease can't ease their pain and suffering or stimulate their appetite by legally growing (or obtaining) and smoking marijuana.

Something stinks here besides that cigarette. Sorry — I couldn't help myself. I'll get back on track.

Anyone who is ill in any way (or healthy, for that matter) and still smoking must not want to live or have any kind of quality of life. My wife felt this statement was insensitive. I feel it's true, and the fact some folks want to quit and can't (or won't) is a further indictment of the smoking habit and the companies that continue to profit from it. And remember who's paying most of the costs (health and labor related to name a few) associated with smoking. Did you know the cost of healthcare in the United States is projected to double in the next ten years? That number is measured in the trillions. At the very least, this paragraph should "ignite" some debate.

A couple of studies say smoking may occasionally be good for this or that.

Gimme a break. Jumping off a high building can be "good" fun, exhilarating, and even "uplifting" until you hit the ground at terminal velocity and turn into a smudge on the sidewalk. No doubt it can "fix" the headache you may have had before you jumped, but ...

I have to believe that there are far better ways to achieve the same potentially positive results of smoking (if such a thing really exists) without risking the mountain of negative ones. Please, don't smoke, ever! And if you're ill, make quitting number one on your list.

Okay, okay, I'll move on.

SLEEP

When you're ill or just in shock from hearing your scary diagnosis, you may not be sleeping well (an understatement, I know).

However, you should allow yourself to sleep as much as you need to. Some of us find it hard to stay in bed, including me.

Here's what I learned about sleep and illness.

Try not to schedule things like doctors' appointments or other meetings in the mornings. After a scary diagnosis, if your symptoms aren't keeping you awake, the constant worrying probably will be. Giving yourself permission to sleep as much as you need to may be easy for some people to do, but hard for others. At first I felt guilty sleeping well into the morning. But given that I was up late stressing, I really needed the rest.

Many of us can't really focus on what's happening to us until everyone else has gone to bed. Nighttime is classically when dark thoughts overwhelm the positive ones. Imagining worst cases makes it really hard to sleep. If you decide to be proactive and start researching your condition(s) and your options, you can scare yourself "sicker" by falling into the trap of focusing on the worst cases.

Even if you gradually teach yourself not to focus on "what if" but instead on what is, and then on what you would like to see happen, the very process of researching your situation, added to other daily activities, will rob you of precious and desperately needed sleep.

Trust me on this one. Your body needs to regenerate. Some of your bodily functions are programmed to happen at night when you're sleeping. They're designed to take advantage of the hours without sunlight and tick along using your body's clock, not the clock on the wall.

You may think you need the "hope" that your nighttime research will bring more than you need sleep. But if you're focused on the right things during your search, you'll soon realize getting enough good quality sleep is an important initial step toward stabilizing your body and thinking clearly — and at the very least toward feeling a bit better.

So what's enough sleep, and what's good quality sleep?

Enough is easy — whatever is enough is for you. Sleep till you wake up naturally. Don't jump right out of bed. Take a minute to breathe and take stock. Forget the averages or theories on whether short naps or marathon sleeps are best. Experiment until you figure out what makes you feel best.

Sleep too much and then cut back a bit. The idea is to feel rested.

Just because your spouse says four hours is plenty doesn't mean ten hours isn't your number. Perhaps some people do best with little sleep, but my experience is most people need more than they can normally get or are willing to admit needing. Some people haven't experienced enough good quality sleep for so long, they wouldn't recognize it if they saw it.

Good quality sleep is restful, uninterrupted sleep. We may be up and down using the bathroom or taking medication or rolling around for any number of reasons. It's important to just do the best you can. That'll look different for each of us and is something we simply need to work at.

Here's another tip.

My wife and I use what we call a "sleep machine." It produces white noise and sounds a bit like rain or a waterfall. In fact it has settings for those sounds. Using a white-noise machine gets you used to a steady environment, sound-wise. My wife says it drowns out my snoring (I think she's hearing the dog, not me — he snores big time). We use it when we travel — it's great in noisy hotels. I find just hearing it gets me thinking about snoozing. Try one. I'm guessing once you get used to it, you won't want to sleep without one.

I've read that the hours of sleep before midnight are way more beneficial than all the hours after midnight. I believe that's true but have yet to achieve the goal of "early to bed." Of course all of this writing and researching doesn't help me get to bed any earlier, but I promise to work on doing just that — once I finish the last chapter of this book.

The rare nights I do get to sleep early seem to result in a more restful and therefore more productive sleep. Remember, it's a process, and for me researching and writing into the night "feels" like more of a priority for me right now. I stay up late and sleep late, but intellectually I know I have some more changes to make. We all need to work on getting to the point where we implement the information we've found relevant and important.

As you begin your own research, remember that last bit. Finding stuff out is step one, but not much happens until you implement some of the items in your plan. Improvement requires taking action. It's hard to change everything overnight.

Because sleep is so important and may be so hard to come by for the variety of reasons noted above, taking a sleeping pill may be a good thing short-term and from time to time. I say this even though, as I think I've made clear, I believe minimizing drug use is probably best and may actually be essential for some of us.

Having said this, I also want to note that there are various teas, herbs, supplements, and other alternatives you may want to try first. I use a variety of things but occasionally sleep is elusive and I allow myself to take a sleeping pill guilt-free — well, almost guilt-free — if I feel I really need to.

EXERCISE

Of course the subject of sleep eases us right into exercise. Regular exercise has an impact on how well and how long we sleep. No doubt exercise may be tough if you're tired from lack of sleep, so this can clearly become a vicious cycle — and not the exercise kind.

Initially, you probably won't be even remotely interested in any kind of exercise. You may feel you're unable to exercise. Both exercise and sleep are important for feeling better and getting better. Both reduce stress and its effects. Both are things you should be focusing on as a priority regardless of where you are in the process of dealing with your health issues.

Obviously, exercise should be given careful consideration depending on your condition and should be discussed with your doctor.

There are all kinds of exercise, and people exercise for all kinds of reasons. The exercise we're going to focus on is basic and targets general health.

If you can't stand, get a cane, a walker, an arm (someone's help) or get yourself into a wheelchair. Do what you can when you can. How you respond, the action you take, is what it's all about.

Let's start with first things first. If you can walk, even a bit, try to walk often. Challenge yourself, but listen to your body. Stress comes in lots of flavors and physical stress needs to be monitored and minimized just like all the other kinds. Walking is good. Walking outside is best. Walk as much as you can and as often as you can and remember to breathe while you walk. Breathe slow and deep.

Do some reading about walking and breathing.

Stretching is good, too. Even if you're stuck in a chair or a bed, you can do a bit of stretching. If you need help, ask for it. Do a search of the Internet using the phrase "stretching in bed." You'll be surprised by what you find.

Yoga, tai chi, and Qigong (also spelled Chi Kung or Chi gong) are just a few of the exercise disciplines with stretching and breathing at their core. It's become easier and easier to find classes or courses offering this kind of exercise opportunity. All kinds of books and tapes are available, too.

Start slow, but start.

Some of it is actually fun. Getting just a little bit of exercise can make a huge difference in your day — and in your night.

We talked a bit about your lymphatic system earlier on. It is important to keep your lymph moving, and getting up and being active will help you do just that.

Since, unlike your blood, your lymph system has no real pump, breathing and moving are important to help your body clean itself up. Many believe cleaning yourself from the inside out is essential to healing. A properly functioning lymphatic system is one of the ways your body detoxes. It's well worth the effort to help that process along any way you can.

Your body also uses sweating, breathing, and elimination as detoxification opportunities. I try to break a sweat once a day. Some good healthy sex is certainly a plus. It may be the furthest thing from your mind, but it may help you in more ways than the obvious ones.

Here's a specific example of how to get things moving and breaking a sweat (no, not that — we've moved on from sex).

A rebounder is a little mini trampoline that you can use inside. A gentle up-and-down motion on it can help you "pump" lymph. We're not talking about doing flips or attempting to bounce your head off the ceiling. We are talking about a gentle bouncing that can include some arm movement, twists, and a focus on breathing. Rebounding gets you moving, breathing, and sweating. It's all good.

Rebounders can be bought with a bit of a railing if you need to hold onto something or steady yourself. I recommend getting it, just in case.

Several companies make rebounders, and some can be folded for easy storage or transport. Rebounders often come with a video describing basic sessions and all kinds of advanced sessions for when you begin to feel better and would like to get more serious.

Since rebounding is a low-impact exercise, it tends to be easy on your body. Based on my reading and experience, I believe you get a good "return" on the effort you put in.

There's something I really like about a rebounder. Even if you can only sit on the thing and have someone else gently bounce on it so you're moving up and down, you're at least getting some benefit — and no doubt it's good for a laugh or two. As we all know, laughing is a very good thing. So even if you're in a wheelchair, you can still make use of a rebounder.

Do an Internet search for "rebounders." There's loads of information and some great testimonials. I'll put some information on my website as well (www.ScaryDiagnosis.com).

Conventional bicycles can be tough on the body, but today there are lots of choices for cycling. There are several flavors of recumbent bikes (often referred to as bents), allowing for easy pedaling in a comfortable and ergonomic position.

These bikes come in three-wheeled versions (trikes), allowing easy riding and great stability even for those with physical or balance-related challenges. Many of the manufacturers of recumbents are small operations and customize bikes and trikes to allow almost anyone to ride regardless of physical limitations.

An example of how customized these bikes can be are the ones set up to be pedaled by hand. If your legs are an issue, this may be the option for you.

When I spoke to one of the recumbent manufacturers, he told me he rides a trike even though he's perfectly healthy and can ride whatever he likes. He said the comfort and stability of a recumbent trike made it more pleasurable to ride.

Many of these bicycles can be rigged up to ride indoors like an exercise bike — in fact, exercise bikes are available in the recumbent configuration. The right kind of bike riding can really be good for your body and overall health.

Getting our lungs working and blood flowing just has to be a good thing for most of us.

It's also good to set some goals and think about riding your bike outside, whether you're capable of it right now or not. Take some slow deep breaths and imagine the outside air running through your hair (yes, I'm assuming you have hair), knowing you're making progress toward your goal. Even just thinking these thoughts is a good thing after a scary diagnosis.

STRESS

Although I've always worked hard — too hard and too much, I now realize — I did take some time to decompress. For years that took the form of fly-fishing, and fishing in general. Today, golf is number one on my list.

Unfortunately, winter is a very unhealthy time for me. I don't really like the cold and therefore don't get nearly as much exercise to keep healthy and reduce stress. Pre-diagnosis, we did do some traveling to warm climates in the winter, but one way or another the travel was typically work-related.

For me, as time passed, work translated directly into major stress and then into all stress all the time. Even when not at work I was always thinking about it or discussing it with my wife or friends (my wife and most of our friends were in the same business).

I still catch myself stressing just thinking about work and work-related issues both past and present. There are pros and cons to having your partner in life also be your business partner. In the past it was, overall, a very good thing for me. Now, however, we've agreed to leave me out of "our" business.

In retrospect, before my diagnosis I had very poor stress-management skills, which probably made me unpleasant to be with at times (to say the least). I am sorry and here and now I apologize to those who knew me then.

Stress is mostly self-inflicted, and a very bad thing. ("No kidding," you're probably thinking.) Moderation is a very important lesson to be learned and is a big part of who I am becoming today. I am "becoming" daily. I'm now a person who (at least most days) takes the time to plan out a more balanced life. That may sound corny, but it comes close to describing how I feel and what I'm doing.

Since what you think can have a very profound effect on your health and wellness, particularly long-term, anything you can do to comfort yourself and those around you has got to be a major plus.

Take the time — give yourself the time — to reflect on what has happened to you and those around you. Have a good look at what your options are as you move forward. Don't dwell too much on why. Focus on now and how, taking things one day at a time. Once you make a plan, look forward, not back.

TWELVE

A NEW ME AND A NEW YOU

The doctor of the future will give no medicine,
but will instruct his patient in the care of the human frame,
in diet, and in the cause and prevention of disease.
— THOMAS ALVA EDISON

AS A RESULT of dealing with my scary diagnosis, I realize more than ever the importance of self-renewal in all its forms — physical, mental and emotional, and spiritual.

PHYSICAL RENEWAL

When I first received my scary diagnosis, I slumped into passivity, fear, and perhaps even a little self-pity. It wasn't long, however, before I decided to take charge of my health and life through research and making my own decisions, both inside and outside the healthcare system. I believe this attitude and the support of my wife, family, and some of my old friends, along with many new ones, are what sparked my self-renewal.

Certainly, on the physical side of things, if I *had* listened to what they were predicting for me at the MS clinic, I might be tapping along with a cane or wheeling about in a wheelchair today, and you definitely *would not* have this book in your hands.

It has been three years since "fuzzy eye." I have no additional attacks to report. No additional symptoms have surfaced. My golf game is improving (although it's not where I'd like it to be, but that's true of all golfers). I feel stronger and more confident about my health every time I swing a club. The important thing is, the numbness in my side and occasional issues with my balance and eyesight are typically not to blame for my variable golf scores. The fact I'm able to play and enjoy physical outings is fantastic, especially considering at the onset of my illness I was told to be prepared to be golf-cart-bound and perhaps even to have to give the game up entirely. (This will only be my tenth season playing — in golf years I'm just getting started.) I'm here to tell you, *do not* listen to all that negative stuff.

I have more feeling in my numb side. I have principally my chiropractor and osteopath, along with my improving physical condition overall, to thank for that. I still believe I will eventually have a "normal" right side. I'll continue to do all I can to that end.

My left arm, whose weakness had extended into my left hand so as to make my pinkie almost useless, has improved significantly. I work on it by continuing to teach myself guitar and doing the exercises that go with it. I've found that as my left hand gets stronger, my golf is getting better. (I had to blame those bad shots on something — any self-respecting golfer will always have at least one excuse at the ready.)

My eye is still a bit fuzzy. It's not that it doesn't focus right; it's still more about processing light and color. On sunny days things get a bit washed-out, and I tend to notice the weakness at dusk. (I'm rarely up in time to see the dawn.) I will say my eye is a bit better than a year ago. Initially I was aware of its being out of whack almost all the time. The human body is certainly amazing and will work to heal itself if you can just limit the bad stuff it has to deal with and help it along when you can. These days, more often than not, I "forget" that my eye isn't working properly.

I have almost no bad days anymore. Low barometric pressure still seems to trigger some symptoms, or at least I tend to notice them more then, but in general I'm feeling good. Really good!

I rarely get sick, as in having a cold or flu. I believe that's a side benefit of my focus on nutrition and of taking LDN. Many LDN users say they have experienced similar reductions in these kinds of illnesses as a "positive" side effect of taking that drug. I also believe lots of vitamin C helps. On the rare occasion that I do get sick, I often seem to get "sicker" than anyone else suffering from the same thing. I guess that's just a new reality I'll need to get used to. In the grand scheme of things, it's no big deal.

I'm again a (more than) healthy 178 pounds, give or take (and if you could take a few, that would be great). I treat myself more often to some of the foods and drinks I chose to avoid completely right after my diagnosis. I try to eat and drink right 80% of the time. Most weeks I'm closer to 90%.

I haven't gotten back into bike riding yet, but I plan to. I wasn't a big bike rider pre-diagnosis, though cycling was my primary means of transportation throughout high school and university. A recumbent bike or trike is still part of my plan. I do walk a fair bit, and when the weather permits I walk 18 holes on the golf course. This next bit is good news and bad news, I suppose, but my yard work once again includes cleaning the eaves troughs, mowing, and cleaning up leaves.

My days often include writing. I plan to continue even after I've completed this book. I still get calls from people wanting help and they remain a top priority for me.

I've helped open a Nutritional Testing Clinic, partly as a result of the testing Dr. Brian Smuk and others put me through regularly. I participate in this business several hours a week. This involvement helps me continue to make good decisions for nutrition, wellness, and therefore life.

Most of all, I relish each and every moment I spend with my wife, family, dog, and friends.

MENTAL AND EMOTIONAL RENEWAL

When I first "went fuzzy," my eye was only part of the problem. My thinking was muddled. To say I was confused is an understatement. The inability to think clearly and that "buzzing" in my head (often mentioned by msers) scared me as much as or more than my eye did.

I remember vividly how frightened I was and how tough it was to get hold of myself. I'm reminded of it every time I speak to someone facing a health crisis. When things are going really wrong health-wise, not being able to think clearly is normal no matter what the health issues may be. That inability to concentrate comes from the shock and awe of the symptoms or diagnosis and can become a prison.

So how does one experience mental and emotional renewal, then?

Getting going quickly was huge for me and definitely contributed to the positive outcome I've enjoyed to date. A quick start means getting past the shock and awe and taking action. You need to get thinking and feeling as soon as possible.

In order to take action that has a chance of some positive results, you need information. You then need to use that information in order to develop a plan. Then it becomes all about implementing, updating, and refining that plan, often daily.

I guess you could say that in the process of renewal, you're using information to create inspiration that will result in transformation (pretty catchy, don't you think? — but oh, so true).

Thinking things through clearly is important, but kind of tough to do if your emotions are fried or buried deep down. I learned I needed to talk about my feelings. In my case I didn't end up seeking professional help (although, if you'll remember, I was game to do so). My wife and others were willing and able to support me. If you need help recognizing and talking about your emotions, get it. You simply must come to terms emotionally with what's happening to you in order to get to the point where you're productively proactive. That's where the power is. That is "empowerment."

These days I'm thinking more and more clearly. That's happening in two ways. First my head rarely buzzes and I am able to read for longer and longer periods of time. Second, I'm calmer and feel more comfortable with what's happening to me. The result is that I remember and can think about more of what I read. At least I seem to be able to do that with material I find interesting or important. The unimportant stuff seems to fly out of my head, but it pretty much always did.

I can play a bit of chess, remember guitar chords, and hold long and often detailed conversations. I'm hoping the people I talk to enjoy these conversations as much as I do.

I'm occasionally asked for my advice on business and life decisions from local business people and friends, which signals to me that, at least for some, I have "rematerialized." I focus my advice on what I've come to really enjoy — big-picture, strategic thinking and generally the more creative side of things.

I feel more focused when I try to help someone follow a pro-active path with their scary diagnosis. That's become an increasingly important part of my life and a measure of where I'm going and to some extent is defining the person I want to be.

SPIRITUAL RENEWAL

Meditation

Personally, I often used to use the terms "meditation" and "prayer" interchangeably.

Whether you view them as two very different and distinct things or as almost the same thing, they can be very helpful and important parts of your "treatment."

Meditation is a very broad subject that ranges from simple to fairly complicated. There are great books and tapes readily available, and courses pop up almost everywhere.

For our purposes let's stay very basic. Start by finding a very relaxed position. Make sure you're comfortable and warm. Use pillows under your head and knees if lying down. Some people prefer to sit. Breathe slow and deep using your belly — in through the nose and out through the mouth. Let things slow down. It is best to have a quiet spot. I use those headphones that cancel out sound and play a soothing "meditation" disc. You can learn all about the "how" by doing an Internet search, buying a book or tape, or taking a class.

The initial goal is to reduce stress, relax, and mentally check in with each bit of your body, starting with your toes. Consciously relax each area as you move up your body. You'll find parts of you are tense that you weren't consciously aware of. Concentrate on slow, rhythmic belly breathing. Be gentle and don't force things. It often takes a bit of practice, but it's worth it.

That's it for meditation. Disappointed because you were just getting interested? Good! There are too many things to discuss and learn about it to spend any more time with it here. My goal is just to get you curious enough to want to learn more and give it a try. I'm betting you'll be happy you did.

Prayer

For me prayer is about taking stock emotionally, being thankful, focusing on the needs of others as well as my own, and talking to and working things through with God. I'll do that my way and you should do it your way.

If you need help in this area you might consider the support most organized (or perhaps commercialized is a better word) religious disciplines offer. Spiritual support and advice are typically available and often a comfort. Since religion is a highly personal subject, we'll stay very general here.

You may choose to do some searching on the Internet, or through books or conversations with others. When things look bad, many turn to prayer and religion. Often people get discouraged too quickly or have a preconceived notion of what answers they may receive or what conclusion they may come to. If they don't get what they want immediately, they move on. Although we typically want to be made healthy or whole instantaneously, it rarely happens that way. Often the lessons learned are subtle and may come from some surprising places or result from something that starts out being considered bad.

I believe spirituality involves personal searching and relationships. Sometimes religion offers that. Other times it seems to have lost its way, getting caught up in politics and power. When you're dealing with a scary diagnosis, working on and contemplating your beliefs can and typically does become part of what you go through. Some people are strong and set in their faith, but many more have deep and often nagging questions. I'm not telling you what to do or how to do it. I'm urging you to do some exploring and give yourself the benefit of the doubt.

I found learning about and thinking about my spirituality and religion, while learning about what others thought and believed as well, opened up some very interesting doors and changed the way I think, act, and feel. I believe this has led to a tangible effect on my illness and certainly changed how I interact with others in the new post-diagnosis world around me.

I also believe I've become a better person as a result of what I've gone through. If that sounds conceited to you, consider that it implies, correctly, that I may not have been such a great person before all this happened.

Before my illness and diagnosis I wasn't very religious. I think of "being religious" as participating in organized or commercialized religion. (I'm sure anyone I've talked to about this is laughing out loud right about now because I'm nothing if not opinionated.) I make no judgments about organized religion. It's not for me to judge as good or bad. Generally there's just too much rhetoric and politics in it for me. My experience, however, has resulted in a heightened awareness of and respect for pretty much all religions, and perhaps more importantly a respect for people's spirituality, which I appreciate as a very good thing indeed.

If an organized religion is already something that's part of your life, embracing and exploring it after hearing your own scary diagnosis will no doubt be helpful to you. If not, some exploration, reading, and discussion may lead you in unexpected directions. I think I always believed in God but tried hard not to think too much about it. However, when there's trouble, most people, even those who aren't religious, tend to pray and contemplate the meaning of life. I certainly did some praying and know that I had lots of people praying for me. Sometimes people say they'll pray for you because they feel it's the right thing to say. In my case I know lots of people really did take the time and make the effort to pray for me, and I believe it was helpful both for them and for me. I read recently that some folks think the power of prayer should be labeled as a subset of Energy Medicine. I think I agree because, at the very least, thinking positive thoughts is way better than thinking negative ones, for every kind of renewal.

So, I'm still not "religious," but I can definitely say I am more aware of and interested in my spirituality. To me this means I know I believe in God, I pray for myself and others, and I appreciate and respect what others choose to believe about God and prayer. There's more to it for me than just that, but that's enough for now.

When it comes to health and wellness and the subject of religion, let's finish by being concerned with the acts of searching and believing rather than with what our individual beliefs may be.

Please use your search engines to have a look at "mind body," "prayer," and "meditation," adding key words that describe your situation.

Please don't overlook or minimize the power that prayer or meditation can have in your health crisis. I truly believe that in addition to the obvious emotional and mental effects, there can be, and often is, a real physical impact as well.

Spiritual changes can take on some interesting forms.

For example, these days my wife and I participate in a dinner club. It consists of four couples of different backgrounds and a couple of different flavors of religion. We get together about once a month. We switch houses and have dinner together (for me including food in such proceedings is always a good thing). At first we discussed a list of questions about religion, faith, and spirituality. Now we've moved into reading some books and discussing them. These things stimulate thoughts, trigger emotions, and keep us focused on relationships and people. I never realized how important those things are and truly believe they can have an impact on your health an every level. Having a "people" and "relationship" focus seems to move us all down the path of appreciating our similarities rather than our differences. This feels like healthy and helpful growth to me.

This club started after my diagnosis and I often wonder how open to it I would have been without that experience.

My scary diagnosis has changed me in so many ways. The illness and diagnosis are slowly becoming just another one of the experiences that make me who I am as a person. It's just another piece of the "me" puzzle. I believe if you're being productively proactive about what's happening to you health-wise, you'll find you too can move past your diagnosis, whether physically, mentally, emotionally, or spiritually. If you work hard at it and are lucky, perhaps you'll move past it in all those ways.

I'd like to close by quoting some of my wife's words about me that I included earlier in the book. I was quite moved, encouraged, and inspired (not to mention a bit surprised) when I read them for the first time. They still choke me up a bit now. If there was this much benefit and potential "good" for a plain vanilla guy like me in my scary diagnosis, I figure there has got to be at least this much for you.

Every day Alan learned more. I honestly feel like he's done a university degree in this subject. I saw him gain strength physically, mentally, and spiritually. He looks healthier and *is* healthier than he was before his diagnosis. He's also more compassionate, sensitive, and patient.

I think things always happen for a reason, or at least that you can use all things for good with the right motivation. I told Alan this diagnosis could be a whole new purpose for him. By helping himself he could help countless others who don't know where to start, or don't know what to do, and that he could not only be compassionate but possibly pave the way for others.

He has done that for many people. Not just people with MS, but those with cancer, colitis, and so much more. He was willing to research anything for anyone because he knew how helpful it could be and how lost people can feel. We don't all have the same gifts and talents, but when we use the ones we have to help others — well, that's truly what it's all about, and I couldn't be prouder of him.

I plan to continue doing my best not to disappoint her, or myself, as time moves along.

In closing, let me say I'm so pleased and thankful for the improvements in my health and the changes in me as a person that I've enjoyed so far. With the help of my wife and others, I've been able to take charge of my health and life in spite of my scary diagnosis.

And you can do this, too. You just need to get started.

There were never so many able, active minds at work on the problems of disease as now, and all their discoveries are tending to the simple truth — that you can't improve on nature.
— THOMAS ALVA EDISON